Passing Through

Recovery from Diabetes and Food Addiction

By Carl Eugene Moore

Cover Art by Jennifer Latini – www.ivareeze.com

Author Photo by Christa Harder – www.christaharder.com

www.carlmoore.org | carlmoore@yahoo.com

passingthroughbook.wordpress.com

ISBN: 978-0-9676837-2-0

Copyright 2011 by DCFX Press – www.dcfx.com

Chapter 1

November 1988

I was driving my mother's new Chevy Spectrum to my first doctor's appointment in years. Autumn in South Carolina was a slow progression from long, humid August days to the chilly mornings and sun-warmed afternoons of November and December. The day was crisp and beautiful with a light blue painted all the way up. The dark tinted driver's side window was down and the cool country air swept past me into the car. I easily filled the fuzzy blue driver's seat well beyond the manufacturer's intended weight limit, my belly overflowing onto the center console. The rust colored satin lining of my XXXL bomber jacket was soft and warm against my thick arms, the brown elastic sleeves stretched tight to accommodate my wrists. I wore short sleeve shirts all year. Layers of fat insulated me from the need to wear a jacket for warmth; the distressed brown leather was all fashion statement. With extra pockets.

Having just turned twenty-one, I was young and strong and indestructible as most college students are. *Merely a precaution*, I kept telling myself, *doing it for Mom to shut her up and get Jill off my back.*

A few weeks earlier, my thoroughly slender friend Jill Diaz and I were crowded in the small Chevy riding around on a Saturday night. We weren't so much on a date as two friends out together and away from our respective college campuses. Not that I wouldn't have been delighted to date Jill, but ours was more an ongoing friendship begun in high school.

"You up for another Mountain Dew?" I asked.

"I haven't finished this one," Jill replied.

I was already on my fourth Dr. Pepper.

All evening I stopped at convenience stores every hour to go to the bathroom and buy yet another soda. My thirst was unquenchable no matter how much liquid I tried to pour on it. Jill put her hand on my arm.

"Carl, something's wrong." I could hear the genuine concern in her voice. "You shouldn't be that thirsty and have to pee all the time. You need to get that checked."

"I'm fine. Just thirsty tonight," I said, brushing her off with practiced casual male bravado. She dropped her protest with a deep, resigned female sigh, but I knew she was right. Something was wrong.

I was keeping very regular bathroom hours including every break between classes and all through the night. My bladder made sure I never got a full night's sleep. My life began to revolve around my next soda and my next trip to the water closet. Over time, I learned the location of every public restroom in Newberry and Greenwood, becoming a regular visitor at several. I could easily take down a twelve pack of Coke, Mountain Dew, or Dr. Pepper in a day; every ounce left me just as quickly.

Jill's concern stayed with me, and I began thinking maybe I was really having health issues. That quiet little voice, however, was lost among the volume of everyday college life.

*

I was attending Piedmont Tech in Greenwood, but basically lived with buddies in their dorm rooms on the Lander College campus across town. Alcohol was ever-present in the small dorm refrigerators; we never seemed to have room for food alongside the carefully maintained inventory of shiny aluminum cans. I followed the beer. Friday and Saturday nights were a steady line of students walking to the Scotsman convenience store just off campus. Underage beer was sweet and easily purchased, brought back on campus by the case. My circle of friends began the party just after classes on Friday afternoon and continued through the weekend. Monday mornings were ritualistic affairs of aspirin and the odd folk remedy.

I indulged my prurient college interests with no small effort. In a weekend, I could easily drink an entire case of cheap beer, cans overflowing the fast food wrapper filled trash bag. There was a Huddle House a short walk from the dorm. We wasted many late nights and early mornings sitting in a booth, drunk and ravenous. We ordered pizza and burgers and hot dogs and chili cheese fries in an endless parade of fat and carbohydrates, washing it down with yet more beer smuggled in our jackets or taped to our legs under jeans.

One morning I woke very early and somewhat disoriented from the inebriated haze generally present on weekends. My right calf hurt. At first, it felt like I had been kicked in the leg. Perhaps I had forgotten the injury while drunk the night before. Then I moved. The pain was intense. I reached down and massaged the spot for a while, drifting back to sleep under the thin blanket. Cramps were common, after all. A few times in high school, I woke to charley horse. Sometimes the morning after a hard football practice, we got them; Coach said we weren't drinking enough Gatorade. So I ignored and forgot about it until the next morning when it happened again. I began having the same pain every morning, and there wasn't football practice or any other kind of exercise to blame it on. Then I began having cramps in both calves at the same time around five in the morning. The discomfort began to hurt enough to jolt me awake. One Sunday, after a night's hard drinking, I woke to intense pain in both calves and both shins at the same time.

That was new.

I couldn't move my foot forward or backward without bolts of searing pain shooting down through my calves and shins. Since I was on the top bunk, rolling out of bed and onto the cold tile floor was a trip I hadn't properly packed for. My buddy and his girlfriend, below me in the bottom bunk, were enjoying a deep, post-alcohol, post-coital sleep, never rousing to notice me falling from the top bunk to lie writhing in pain on the cold, white tile floor.

The cramping pulled my leg muscles into knots.

I was able to roll onto my stomach and slowly crawl up the bedpost. I stood hugging the bunk bed's grey metal post for several minutes until the cramping passed. The soreness stayed with me the rest of the day. Several subsequent painful mornings finally prompted me do something.

I called the doctor's office and talked with a nurse about my symptoms. She said I needed to make an appointment for a checkup. Easy enough. I expected to walk in, let them poke and prod me, and I would be on my way. The cramps would pass, of course. With time, they always had. Maybe I had been drinking a little too much or shoveling down a few too many chili cheese fries.

I was a growing college boy, of course, and these things were normal, expected. There was this little voice of doubt, though, that said maybe I needed to take the situation a little more seriously, but I was never one to listen to little voices. I liked my voices loud, punctuated with profanity.

*

The small brick building was once the only in the area. The six bed private hospital was hidden by foliage left unrestrained for years. The doctor's office could have easily been built before the war. The Civil War. The entire building blended quietly into the surrounding woods off the two-lane highway just outside downtown Prosperity, South Carolina.

The longtime physician in residence matched the structure. He may have actually been a field surgeon dressed in a threadbare grey wool uniform treating wounded on the field. He was so ancient and infirm himself that he seldom left an equally antique high-backed wooden chair in his office. Instead of going to the exam room to see patients, he had them come in turn into his tiny, paper-stacked office to be examined. Usually his nurse, also his much younger wife, did most of the clinical work, consulting him for a signature on a prescription pad. I had been an overnight guest in the hospital when I was five or six and remembered even back then his movement was more tortoise than hare.

As I passed the train tracks leading into Prosperity, I saw the town's day shift police officer sitting in his patrol car, black radar gun in hand. I had seen the blue, rotating dome light enough that year to respect the posted thirty-five limit.

The gravel and dirt parking lot was small with only a few cars in it. I pulled into the lot, parked, and began the process of emerging from the snug cocoon of the compact car. I was so large that the small car felt more like a big, metal overcoat than conveyance; I was a hermit crab shrugging off his shell in search of a new one. Just getting in meant folding backward into the metal doorframe and plopping into the driver's seat. I often joked I might forget one day to get out of it and wear the car inside.

Some of the tall bushes surrounding the brickwork would require a chainsaw to tame, while kudzu vines threatened to pry torn screens from all the paint-peeled windows. I found the vine-covered wrought iron railings and the long, inclined concrete ramp to the door. There was something ominous about the long walk, like the last walk a death row prisoner takes after the last meal and last rites have both been observed. Even the dozen or so feet up the ramp started sweat running down the back of my black t-shirt. I shrugged out of the leather jacket tossing it causally over my shoulder.

A wide, heavy wood door at the end of the walkway was painted in several dozen coats of white oil paint with various shades showing through as cracks peeled up from the layers underneath. The antique fixtures had long since turned a malicious shade of green. When I grasped the handle, I cringed ever so slightly, perhaps feeling that some of the green might wipe away and become embedded in the ridges of my chunky fingers. To be as heavy as it was, though, the door swung effortlessly on its hinges, emitting a loud squeal as if it were to a castle dungeon. Three or four faces turned to me. My embarrassed smile answered them before everyone went back to doing the nothing people do sitting in a waiting room.

I looked around to find the interior was larger than it looked from outside, almost cavernous, and smelling of "simmering grandmother," a pairing of moth balls and formaldehyde. I remembered the smell from my stay as a child. The decor reminded me of a train station or art deco restaurant out of the 1920s with the high ceilings, white walls, black trim, and alternating black and white floor tiles. Doric columns were spaced throughout the room, simple scrollwork adorning each where it joined the ceiling. There were no chairs, rather simple bench seats around the exterior of the room, small end tables with marble tops held magazines and black deco lamps with clear, low wattage bulbs. The curtains were heavy, dreary affairs in dark colors gathered at the windows with large gold ropes.

"Can I help you?"

I recognized the receptionist's voice from when I called for the appointment. She sat in an adjacent room behind a small counter shelf and window separating her from the waiting area. She was a pretty woman, lightly tanned, perhaps in her mid thirties, with full brown hair down past her shoulders. She had a pleasant, but occupied look about her, even though the waiting room wasn't exactly full and it was still early.

"I have an appointment," I said walking toward her.

"Name?"

"Carl Moore. I have an 8:30."

"Yes," she said, finding my name on her sheet like a warden scrolling down a list of trusties requesting a conjugal visit. "Sign in, please." She indicated a clipboard with names already scribbled on it. A thin, black pen with a long, silver beaded chain lay on the counter. I wondered who would want to steal such a cheap pen. I wrote my name and the time on the next available line.

"Yes, Mr. Moore, we want to get a fasting blood sugar on you," she said as she moved papers on her desk. When I had called, the nurse told me, "That means you fast from midnight the previous night until you get into the office and we can run the test. Don't eat anything after midnight before coming in or you will throw off the reading. Do you understand?"

Of course I understood. I was a college man, high school graduate, strong as the proverbial ox, and twice as mean. My buddies and I would get a little tanked and pick up small cars in the parking lot and turn them around for fun.

"Yes," I had said and hung up.

Did I understand?

"Are you fasting today," the receptionist asked.

"Yes, ma'am," I replied.

"Good, then we can get labs on you today. Please take a seat and they'll call you back shortly," she said looking up at me with a pretty smile.

I thanked her and took a seat on one of the benches. The magazines on the end table were all out of date. I picked up a *Popular Mechanics* from the previous year and flipped through it looking at the pictures and pretending to read.

The nurse, also the doctor's wife my mom had told me, finally came to the door and called my name. She was severe, not particularly attractive, and obviously devoid of the ability to smile. The white cap, white patent leather shoes, and requisite starched white uniform wore her perfectly. When I rose, she motioned me to come, so I followed her through the door to an area with a long, white counter filled with all manner of medical equipment and supplies. I could feel the nervousness crawl slowly up my back into my neck to tickle the tiny hairs against my black t-shirt. She led me to the most dreaded piece of medical equipment on the planet – the doctor's office scale.

"Up there," she said in monotone, indicating the scale.

I stepped on the black, wobbly platform. The right side of the balance beam leapt into the air. I noted the sour look from the corner of my eye. She reached around me and moved the larger weight one huge click. Then another. Then another. She then slid the smaller weight to the right until the balance beam regained its sanity, wavering almost imperceptibly with my heartbeat as I realized I was holding my breath. Perhaps I thought the extra oxygen would tip the scales somewhat more in my favor.

"Three hundred eighteen pounds," she said in her annoying monotone. She would have been quite at home announcing train arrivals and departures.

She scribbled something in health care hieroglyphics on her clipboard.

"Take a seat," she said, indicating a steel-topped stool, then left me wait alone.

I sat, my butt warming cold metal, and waited for her to return. I was still holding the *Popular Mechanics* from the lobby, though it seemed to have picked up moisture from somewhere. The cover was damp. I wiped my hands absently on my blue jeans and flipped through the magazine while I waited, actually reading most of an article on washing machine repair before the nurse returned.

I didn't own a washing machine.

"We're checking your blood sugar today, correct," the nurse said, more statement than question. Her voice was loud and startled me. I struggled to bend down to pick up the magazine I had dropped.

"Yes, ma'am," I answered grunting as I straightened.

"And you haven't eaten since midnight last night." Statement.

"No, ma'am. I had something around nine last night."

"Good. This is a fasting blood sugar test and we need to do that on an empty stomach. You didn't drink anything this morning." Statement.

"No ma'am," I said, quite conscious of the growing discontent behind my belly button. The ride back to the house was going to be a long one, but McDonalds did, after all, have a drive-through.

She pulled another steel stool from under the counter and sat directly in front of me, her knobby knees pressed against my plump ones, then roughly took hold of my left hand. She had the bedside manner of a diesel stump grinder, and had obviously just come from working the metal handle on an aluminum ice tray.

Maybe more than one.

Turning my palm up, she isolated the index finger with her chilly, bony hands. In one swift stealth attack, she plunged a sharp, steel-tipped lancet into the tender pad of my finger. I jumped and yelped and tried to snatch my arm back, but she held my wrist with all the tenderness of a pro wrestler in the ring, her opponent dazed and bent over the ropes.

Perhaps I had expected Audrey Hepburn in *The Nun's Story*; a soft, pretty face, delicate manners, quiet disposition, and an excellent bedside manner.

This nurse wasn't Audrey.

She squeezed my bleeding finger to get a large drop of dark crimson. Blood pooled there, my life liquids leaking from my body, my skin invaded by the sharp metal I would come to know intimately in later years. Then she took a small cardboard strip about the size of a paperclip, and smeared a large drop of blood on it. When she was satisfied she had enough of my life on the little strip, she released me.

I was bloody.

My index finger was covered in a color I never wanted to see come from me. The wet strip went into a palm-sized blood glucose meter that beeped once. The nurse reached for the gleaming lid of a glass jar in front of her. She extracted a fluffy white cotton ball and passed it to me. I took it and pressed my finger into it. My damaged finger throbbed against the softness.

The meter took several minutes to spin and whirr and calculate the amount of glucose swirling around in my bloodstream. I thought about my last meal, the large green salad with the liquid cardboard fat free dressing and Tab cola I had for dinner the previous evening was not my usual fare of fat, carbohydrate, sodium, and cholesterol, softened by yeast's liquid gifts to man and womankind.

Certainly, the shock to my system could throw off my normal readings. I remembered the nurses' admonition to fast. I never understood why they called it fasting when it was so damn slow.

The blood glucose meter finally beeped again – several beeps this time. Beeping was seldom a good sign coming from anything, especially not in medical equipment. I could see the nurse's sour look curdle.

"Did you know you were diabetic." She wasn't asking.

Diabetic?

Adrenaline's liquid heat bolted through my arteries. I was suddenly flushed, dizzy. I was just out of high school, college and career and a full life ahead of me. Diabetic? That's what grandma got when she was eighty. I couldn't have diabetes. I was too young, too strong.

"No," I finally coughed out weakly, disbelief and fear rising like a toilet on the verge of overflowing.

She looked at me in her passive, condescending, matter-of-fact way and stated, "Well, lose some weight and stop eating sugar." She got up, turned, and left me to sit there and try to get my mind around the revelation that I had a chronic disease at twenty-one.

Chapter 2

July 2007

The afternoon was Southern hot and Southern humid. Initially I parked in the wrong parking garage, had to call someone, get back in my car, find the garage I was supposed to be in, drive up ten heat-radiating, pre-stressed concrete floors, then find my way to the conference room I was supposed to be speaking in. My long sleeve white cotton Old Navy shirt was disturbingly wrinkled by the time I arrived, four minutes from the advertised start time.

The room was smaller than I had expected, a typical corporate meeting room filled with milling, chatting people. Folding chairs were set before a large projection screen in the front of the room; a snack table laden with spiral cut ham attracted a purposed crowd in the rear. The dead pig on the table struck me as ironic for a weight loss group, but I supposed the absence of biscuits and the abundance of Diet Coke made "the other white meat" a diet plate.

I smiled and moved through the mass of talking, eating people towards a thin, pretty blonde lady I supposed was the organizer, Amy. She saw me a few rows deep and we exchanged a smile and nod of recognition as I found my way to the podium she was standing near.

"You must be Carl," she said, extending a small hand.

"I hope so," I said, "I'm wearing his underwear."

She laughed then told me about the order of events.

"We have four people presenting today. All of you have lost at least twenty-five pounds and saw great results with their blood sugars, just like you. One is a nurse who works here at the hospital. Two others are patients who we've treated here recently. One of them, a guy and his dog, drove all the way from Rock Hill to be here today. He's got a wonderful story of just getting out and walking his dog after he was diagnosed. Elizabeth told me you started out doing a lot of walking."

I nodded. "Yes, at first all I did was walk. The first twenty or so pounds just walked themselves off that way. Well, that and I stopped eating Chinese buffet every day."

"Oh, I do love Chinese food," she said. I looked at the skinny woman in front of me expecting she had no chance at getting her money's worth at any buffet in the country, Chinese or otherwise.

At one hundred twenty five pounds lost, I was the heavyweight, as it were, she told me, and would go last and have the longest time to speak, something like thirty minutes. I thought about the thirty-five slides in my presentation knowing I could easily fill an hour or more just covering the material therein. Thirty minutes was seldom enough time for me to explain anything of substance.

"Sure," I said, "I'll try to fill the entire time."

Speaking to the weight loss and diabetes group hadn't been my idea. A month earlier, a coworker set the stage without consulting me.

"You might get a call from Amy Pope at Baptist," Elizabeth emoted, twirling into my office, soft grey cashmere and golden silk fluttering around our tall, thin departmental social butterfly. She flitted through life, lighting here and there, spreading her fifties, sophisticated, girl-next-door charm, educating anyone she could get to stop and listen about diabetes. One of the Certified Diabetes Educators in our practice, Elizabeth, "Miss Eliza Beth," as I called her, knew the disease personally from a young age, having been diagnosed with Type 1 Juvenile diabetes, insulin-dependent at the age of seven in 1959.

Diabetes education back then was non-existent. She learned to check her blood sugar with the archaic tools available and give herself insulin injections with huge, metal syringes that had to be boiled for sterilization between uses.

"And why would I get a call from an Amy Pope at Baptist?" I asked without looking away from my monitor. I had a well-practiced method for entertaining Miss Eliza Beth without being distracted or caught up in her childlike enthusiasm for virtually everything.

"Well," she began in dramatic breathlessness, placing both palms on my desk and leaning in, perhaps to ensure I got the full import of her message. "I told her all about your amazing transformation and she needs speakers for her weight loss and diabetes support group and I know how much you enjoy talking to people about your journey and I just knew you would love to go and speak to her group and she's very excited and can't wait to talk to you about it and you're just perfect for what she needs and you're so motivating and…" she trailed off to take a deep breath. I turned my head enough to look at her over my dollar store reading glasses, replying before she could get enough air to get wound up again.

"So basically you volunteered me for something without bothering to ask me about it first, is that it?"

"No. Well, yes. Well, it's just that…"

I let her fidget a little before giving her my full attention and saying, "Sure, I'd love to talk to their group." I so enjoyed the banter with someone who knew the game.

*

I handed over my flash drive to a technician who set up my slide presentation on the computer in the podium and made sure the first slide was up and ready to advance. The other four speakers came in and we shook hands and exchanged greetings and settled into our seats. Folding chairs always felt unsteady to me and sitting on one close in between other people before an audience was somewhat unnerving. Someone said that civilized man's worst fear is public speaking. After losing as much weight as I had, my biggest fear was not being seen and heard and acknowledged, so I wasn't nearly as nervous as perhaps I should have been.

Amy stood and got everyone's attention. Opening remarks were offered, sponsors were acknowledged, including the ham provider, and the first speaker stood and presented his story. Each in turn related how simple changes in eating habits and lifestyles and an increase in exercise resulted in significant weight loss and a resulting positive effect on their blood sugar levels. All began with high blood sugar levels that had dropped radically once exercise became habit and ten percent or more of their body weight had been shed. Each gave testimony to what diet and exercise could do for a person. Then it was my turn.

"We have with us today someone who has lost one hundred and twenty-five pounds," Amy said to a quiet audience that began to murmur in tones suggesting a mixture of disbelief, awe, and praise. Even those who shared the stage with me gave me their attention.

I stood and took ownership of the room, looking directly into the eyes of each person seated in the front row before beginning.

"I've been wrestling with this shirt all day," I said indicating my wrinkled shirt, "and obviously getting nowhere. So, against advice, I'm just going to untuck and go with what works." I pulled my shirt out of my waistband as a few people golf-clapped and acknowledged the lost battle.

"That's better," I said, moving a bit to get a feel for the area I had to work in.

"I used to be what my mother calls a 'Bad Diabetic'," I began, "I've always been fat, was born a chubby boy. I've lost a lot of weight and I've still got a long way to go to reach my goals, but I'm thirty-nine and in better shape than when I was nineteen."

Support and clapping came to me from all sides as the message began to settle over my audience.

"I was diagnosed as diabetic when I was twenty-one. Twenty. One." I let the words hang in the air for a moment. "That's way too young to be told you have a lifelong, chronic disease that will slowly kill you, slowly take away your eyesight, slowly take away your ability to walk, slowly, painfully take away your quality of life." Heads nodded. If I had been in a Baptist pulpit, I knew an "Amen" or two would have found its way from the back of the room.

I spun the sarcasm knob hard right for effect. "And you know, at twenty-one, I was SO concerned about the diagnoses, SO impressed by the level of diabetes education that I received, that I did absolutely nothing about it for eighteen years." I gave that a moment. "Yeh, the nurse told me I was diabetic and that I needed to lose some weight and quit eating sugar."

I saw heads nod; there was something akin to approving laughter coming from people wrestling with the same issues. I had already connected with my audience and they were ready to take the journey with me. I nodded to a man standing against the wall across from me. As he reached back and lowered the lights, I clicked the handheld slide advancer to the first slide.

Chapter 3

I don't remember the nurse taking me by the hand and leading me back to the front of the doctor's office. I was back in the car and driving home even before I realized I had left. I had written and handed over a check for the visit, stumbled through the waiting room, and found the car in a hazy blur.

Diabetes.

All I really knew about the disease was that it was something old people got later in life, not young, healthy, ox-strong college men with their futures an un-trod carpet rolled out before them. Maybe the nurse was mistaken. Maybe the test results were off; certainly, that kind of thing happened all the time. The blood test wasn't exactly done under ideal, controlled laboratory conditions. Besides, I didn't feel Diabetic.

I had heard the word often enough, of course. I knew I had what doctors called a "family history." My mother always said her mother was a "Bad Diabetic." I sarcastically assumed that when she was younger, she fed her sugar habit by holding up candy stores with her used insulin needles. Those early reusable metal syringes were, after all, nasty-looking affairs more resembling torture devices from the Middle Ages rather than delicate, life-saving medical tools. My family had a dubious history at best. Mom had diabetes at some time in her life, but she claimed that a preacher at a faith healing tent meeting laid hands on her and cured her. I didn't see any old time faith healing tents on the side of the road as I drove.

*

When I got home, I went straight to the kitchen. There was nothing like a white bread, mayo, and cheese sandwich to calm the nerves. So, I had two of them, just in case.

Mom was at work.

My mother had always been old, old and imbued with the strength that comes from the Atlas-like labor of carrying a family on her bent shoulders. The long and troubled southern road she had traveled through the Depression and Second World War showed in cartographic lines etched deeply into the soft tissues of her dark face. Every picture of her looked like an old sepia photograph of Sitting Bull posing on the plains, his favorite Winchester repeating rifle in his weathered hands. She was old even when her hair was a rich sable and full and I was a plump toddler in a kiwi green jumpsuit she had made for me on an old Sears sewing machine, bought "on time." She was over fifty when she adopted me, the eight-year-old only child of her divorcing daughter. Having a grandmother for a mother meant I was spoiled from the outset. When we went to the grocery store, I would snag a pack of hot dogs while we were shopping and I would eat them all before we got to the register where she would hand the clerk the empty package.

A few years later, she endured her own divorce and reentry into a job market unfriendly to a longtime housewife, but she went back to work with no education and after years of working in the mill and did what was necessary to keep me fed and clothed and in school. She took menial, tedious jobs, working third shift in a local nursing home and sitting with patients in the hospital or in the patient's home. She was a kind of nurse who stayed with elderly patients, usually those suffering from Alzheimer's. The patient's family needed help or simply didn't want to be bothered until it was time for the reading of the will, so Mom stayed with them until they died. Often she would stay full time, taking a few hours off every couple of days to take care of things at home, pay bills, buy groceries, and cook, leaving days of leftovers for me in the fridge. Being a caretaker for someone else's family member was a harsh way to make most of a living. Just under five feet and scarcely a hundred pounds, helping the elderly and infirm in and out of bed and pulling at them left her worn and exhausted in the short time she actually spent at home. My mother was a workaholic grown of financial necessity.

Born on Columbus Day in 1923, my mother was also something of a founding member of the "I love you, eat this" generation. Having grown up in the midst of the Depression, then the rationing of World War II, Mom found a way to stretch her earnings to keep food in the house; her pantry was a well-stocked mini A&P. An accomplished and prolific cook before she went back to work, she coated everything in flour or cornmeal and tenderly fried it brown in lard or bacon grease. Gravy, be it brown, white, redeye, or sawmill, was considered a beverage in our house. We ate like field hands, plentiful southern meals dressed richly in creams and sauces and real butter, sided with piles of homemade biscuits and cornbread.

We lived in what used to be called a trailer before "mobile home" and "manufactured housing" entered the marketing vernacular, a phrase invented to make aluminum rectangles sound more attractive as homes. Our twelve foot by seventy-four foot metal home was too hot in August and too cold in February, but I never realized we were poor, testament to my mother's labors.

*

I had skipped Friday morning classes for the doctor's appointment; I could swing by Mom's work in the evening and tell her. I put the books for my afternoon classes in my charcoal-grey plastic Samsonite briefcase and got back in the car. The drive to school was about forty-five minutes on a two-lane road if I didn't get behind a sluggish yellow school bus or lumbering logging truck.

I was attending Piedmont Tech majoring in business. I was able to carry a double class load by taking day classes in Greenwood and taking night classes three days a week at a satellite campus near my home in Newberry. Where class attendance was not requisite, I wandered in for the pre-test reviews and took tests. Since I wasn't working, maintaining a B average was easy enough even with the slight exertion I was putting into it. Weekends were when I expended serious effort, though not in anything as prosaic as academic interests. Weekends were, after all, for partying and I had to conserve my energy.

Classes that afternoon passed unnoticed. The word "Diabetes" seemed to keep appearing in the chalk scratched on every blackboard. I was paying even less attention than usual. After my last class was over, a friend asked me if I would be around for the weekend. I lied, telling him I had things to do at home. I didn't want to answer questions. I decided I would wait to see Mom, too. Diabetes was terminal, I thought.

Saturday morning I slept late. When I did get up, I stopped by the bathroom, then went straight to the kitchen. After filling the copper tea kettle and setting it on the stove to heat, I tore open six packets of instant grits, poured each one into a large bowl, put two pieces of bread in the toaster, and waited to see if the kettle or the toaster would be ready first. The smell of warm toast filled the air. The kettle started to whistle just before the toaster popped.

Cheese and real churned butter turned my Jethro Bodine bowl of hot grits a shade of orange almost matching the large glass of juice I had poured. Mom knew someone in town who churned real butter and sold it in round, pale yellow pint blocks that had flower designs molded into them from the pattern in the bottom of the mold. We kept several of the butter blocks wrapped in wax paper in the refrigerator and freezer. I cut generous portions from a chilled block of the yellow dairy goodness. Using the toast like a spoon for the grits, I ate through the first two pieces quickly, reloaded the toaster and poured more juice.

Breakfast in our house had always been a large, ritualistic affair. Weekdays mom would wake me early so I would have time to eat a large plate of cheese grits, sausage, eggs, and toast before the bus came. My mother was from the generation that showed their love by cooking large, southern meals that generated generous leftovers for days. Even as poor as we were, our pantry shelves always bowed with plenty and our refrigerator was filled with glass gallon bottles of milk and orange juice, blocks of Reagan cheese, and logs of beef bologna. We ate like lumberjacks preparing for the day's work.

*

When I finished eating, I put the dishes in the sink, and took the last of my orange juice with me to the couch to watch Saturday morning cartoons until noon. We got four channels on the tornado-damaged Channel Master antenna, and our television was too old to have a remote control, so I sat on the television end of the couch so I could reach out and change channels.

*

When I was eight or nine years old, I used to walk to the Newberry County library downtown several days a week with a neighbor who walked his dog, Boy. He loved that old dog as much as he would have his unborn children. Boy was a large Labrador with a quiet, gentle disposition, and I enjoyed the walks downtown, the big yellow dog leading, stopping to sniff and mark regularly. The neighbor had long since moved to Florida, sending news a few years later of Boy's death. We learned the neighbor died shortly thereafter. I hadn't wandered into the library or, for that matter, walked any considerable distance since childhood.

After the cartoons went off and the Saturday afternoon replacement window and vinyl siding commercials came on, I got up and fixed two sandwiches and sweet tea for lunch. I wanted more information on the disease, wanted to know what was happening inside me. I owned a computer, but the Internet was still years away from being an instant source of information. I needed the library.

When I finished, I shrugged into my leather jacket, then drove to the library and its sepulcher-like quiet. Some notion of the Dewey Decimal System had stayed with me from high school. One teacher my junior year assigned us a couple of term papers requiring library searches. From those I had a passing familiarity with the card catalog index, though in practice more from a fiction angle than real research. My taste in literature was swords and sorcery fantasy. I went in, found the large, wooden card catalog, opened a drawer, and started flipping through typed index cards.

"May I help you?" a strong, old, female voice asked.

Startled, I glanced left to see a tiny woman of perhaps three hundred years old, considered a giant, I supposed, among her people, the Garden Gnomes. Thick, round glasses protected most of a tiny face, the skin taut on her ancient bones, as if purposefully stretched there for drying. She was dressed plainly, pragmatically against the November chill.

"Diabetes," I said turning to her with my right hand still in the card drawer I had been thumbing through. She didn't blink behind her giant lenses. "I'm looking for books on diabetes. I'm diabetic," I said almost apologetically.

I had a quiet illness with a stigma attached. Certainly, diabetes didn't garner the flavor of prejudice that something like mental illness had, but there was palpable, demonstrable discrimination. I had heard of diabetics losing or not getting jobs. The librarian's face softened, showing me sympathy her voice didn't.

"Well, now, let's see," she said moving toward me. Something about her carriage made me think she could brush me aside if she wanted. I slid my hand out of the drawer and backed away from the huge wooden card catalog case that smelled like musty history.

"Diabetes. That would be 616.462. Here," she said, tapping with one of her short, thin fingers near the drawer I had opened. Her knowledge of Mr. Dewey was intimidating, even a bit frightening. She pulled the long, wooden drawer open and started flipping through the white cards.

"What are you looking for exactly?" she asked over her shoulder.

"Not sure. I was just diagnosed."

"Hmm. Do you use insulin?"

"No, ma'am. They told me not to eat sugar and that I needed to, uh, lose some weight."

"Ah, then you would have adult onset." She cast the fact into the air above her as she continued to flip through cards, examining each one more slowly as she went.

"This should be helpful," she said finally as she conjured a pencil stub and a small, spiral notebook. She wrote on the notepad, closed the drawer quickly, turned, and walked away from me. I lurched into motion to follow. She was quick, like a spooked ferret, and I had to hustle to keep up as she turned left down a tall row of books. When I made the turn, she was walking slowly and looking up, her right hand following some invisible line running across the books. Then her hand stopped as she reached up on her toes to retrieve a small, yellow hardback from the shelf. Her right index finger traced the square spine and lettering before she turned and extended the book to me. I took it.

"That should help you," she said, "come back when you have read it." I felt the command as she breezed past me. I didn't even bother to look at it as I turned to follow. I walked to the checkout desk and handed the book and my blue, cardboard library card with the metal plate identifier number on it to the young girl. She was wearing a grey t-shirt with "Newberry College" in dark red letters screen printed across her chest. She took the white index card from inside the back cover, scribbled down my information, then handed me back the book and card.

"That's due back in two weeks," she said without looking at me.

I stuck the card in my pocket, slipped the book into my leather jacket, and went back out into the afternoon. When I got home, I went to my room and dropped my heavy jacket into a chair. When I tossed the book onto the grey sheets of my queen-sized waterbed, it slid across the slick material like a granite curling stone on ice, skipped over the padded brown vinyl railing, and onto the floor with a carpeted thud. I spun up Steely Dan's Aja album on the turntable. After retrieving the small hardback, I flopped across the moving bed to read.

The word "Diabetes," it turned out, was coined by Aretaeus of Cappadocia in the first century A.D. and translated roughly as "passing through" or "siphon." Apparently, the Greeks must not have had a better word meaning "Pee Your Life Away." I was well aware of that particular symptom of the disease, regular trips to the bathroom.

What I didn't know was that all those potty breaks meant I was losing potassium in record quantities. A low potassium level was the cause of my severe leg cramps. That was useful information, something the doctor could have easily told me, and something that would have made a real difference. Diabetes, after all, didn't hurt; the symptoms were the painful part. I folded the front cover flap in for a bookmark, got up, turned off Steely Dan, and went straight to the A&P grocery store at Eckerd's Square. There I found potassium supplements in the vitamin section. I bought a bottle and a Diet Coke and swallowed two of the round, white tablets in the car, easily finishing off the cold soda. In the coming days, the leg cramps would decrease in severity and frequency until they completely disappeared.

I didn't leave the house Saturday night, but I didn't watch television. I played one album after another: Phil Collins, Genesis, Pink Floyd, Jackson Browne. I continued reading about diabetes, specifically adult onset, or Type 2 diabetes. The information was both compelling and engrossing in the way a multi-vehicle accident is on the road. Even though I didn't want to know, I had to know, so I read on, finishing the book sometime in the small hours of morning.

I had lost a few pounds even before the 318 pounds on the doctor's office scale, and I was even proud of that fact. What I didn't realize was that the weight loss had nothing to do with dieting or exercise, which I took care to avoid. The minor decrease in my weight was due solely to Diabetic Ketoacidoses, a condition that occurs when blood sugar levels are very high and the body begins to break itself down, ergo the weight loss. My blood sugar level was so high that I was literally peeing the weight off in a very unhealthy way not realizing what was happening. My dreams that night reflected my new knowledge. In one, I was standing in front of the porcelain and slowly turning into a huge prune-like thing as I kept flushing, the toilet filling to the rim over and over again.

I tried to sleep between troubling dreams, but after hours of rolling back and forth on the warm waterbed, and several trips to the bathroom, I got up around five and took a hot shower. I would see Mom later in the day and would have to tell her about the doctor's visit.

Sunday breakfast was another festival of grits and toast soaked in real, hand-churned butter, sloshed down with lots of orange juice from concentrate. The clear glass gallon containers of juice never lasted long in our house. After breakfast, I moved to the living room to watch Charles Kuralt for a while, then I got a hot shower and put on something comfortable.

Mom came home after noon when the family she was staying with got home from church and gave her a much-needed couple of hours off. She seemed to know already that I was diabetic, perhaps from her own experiences, but her strategy for coping with things was avoidance or redirection. She started to tell me stories of her mother's history of diabetes. Pictures of my great grandmother from that time showed a large, imposing woman in height and attitude, with deep Native American roots, Comanche or Cherokee from what I was told. She may have actually grown up on a reservation, the youngest, with at least two sisters who were diabetic, as well. She ate whatever she wanted, never exercised, and may have eventually died of diabetic complications the same as her mother had years earlier. I was too young to know much of her, but I remembered her walking out into her back yard, grabbing up chickens, one in each massive hand, and wringing their necks, then letting them go to run around the yard until they died. She would plunge the dead chickens in a large aluminum wash pot of hot water on the back steps, the stench of wet feathers rising. After soaking the dead chicken for a few minutes, she would pull the feathers away from the wet, pink skin before taking the plucked bird inside to fry in an enormous cast iron pan of hot grease. The resulting mounds of deep fried chicken would be surrounded by huge bowls of mashed potatoes with veins of churned butter running through them, white gravy made with pot liquor from the chicken, sweet corn, green beans with bacon or fatback, and a pone of cornbread the size of a large pizza four inches thick with a light, golden crust. Cooking, especially Sunday dinner, was a serious undertaking. With her records indicating two different birth dates, whoever made the decision on her death certificate split the difference and said she was seventy.

Mom stayed for about an hour then went back to work. I spent the rest of the day on the couch alternately eating cheddar and sour cream potato chips and Cheetos and watching Clint Eastwood movies sponsored by a vinyl siding and replacement window company. Sometime that evening I went to sleep, waking up to a test pattern on the television and the unwavering tone that said the station was off the air for the night. I got up and turned it off, went to the fridge, drank some cold whole milk, and went to bed.

Monday morning I got in the car and consulted Ronald McDonald. I pulled up to the drive-through and ordered my usual breakfast on the road – two Sausage and Egg McMuffins with extra cheese, two orders of hash browns, and two orange juices. I was, after all, as my mother always said, a growing boy. I had just read about how bread and potatoes spike blood sugar, but I was hungry and Ronald was accommodating.

After morning classes, I drove to the Lander campus, parked, and went looking for Jill Diaz. She was working as a receptionist in the college's ROTC department as a work-study student. There wasn't much work to the job and even less studying, so we would sit and chat when I visited. Jill's grades were well below average with no hope in sight. I found her sitting at a desk with a teen magazine open in front of her. On the page she was reading, Pat Benatar was wearing something with black leather and white lace. I dropped into a chair and we chatted about our respective weekends. A small radio in a corner was tuned to WBBQ out of Augusta and eighties pop tunes played low in the background. The place smelled like the fusty oil paint slowly extricating itself from the walls and molding. I sat back and listened until it came time for what I dreaded telling her.

"I went to the doctor Friday," I said, hesitating. She let the magazine fall flat on the desk. I had her full attention.

"And?" Her tone was both question and demand.

"Well," I held the moment as long as I could, "they said I have Diabetes." I trailed off when my mouth formed the word.

"Oh, no," she said. Her dark, Hispanic eyes grew wide and she brought her hand up to her mouth. "What do you do?" I realized she didn't know any more about the disease than I did.

"Well," I said, holding back again, "they told me to lose weight. And I have to stop eating stuff with sugar in it," I added, almost as an afterthought.

Her hand dropped to her lap. She paused a second. I could see her working through what I had just dumped on her. Then her face changed.

"What about beer?"

The girl knew me well.

"I dunno," I said seriously, "hadn't really thought of that."

Beer was, I considered, a product of fermentation, meaning sugar was involved. Alcohol hadn't actually been a topic in the book I had just read. Jill had already moved on.

"You know I love you just like you are, but you could lose some weight. I know you've always been a big boy, but that can't be healthy. This will get better if you lose weight, right?"

"So I gather."

"Then do it. I don't want you sick," she said. I knew she meant it.

"Thanks. I'm going to work on it," and I thought I actually would. "I've got a book from the library," I said, pulling it from my jacket. "I read it Saturday night and it's got some good stuff in here. I'd like you to read it," I said extending it to her.

The information in it, quite honestly, had scared me. Diabetes wasn't really talked about, and all the potential complications I read of were nothing I wanted. I wondered why no one had ever told me about Diabetes, why there wasn't some class in high school. Why hadn't the school nurse pulled me aside after homeroom one day and told me that being a lard ass could make you Diabetic? I assumed Jill would want to know, want to learn all that I had, be there to help me, her friend for so many years.

Jill took the offered book and flipped through it. She stopped on a page.

"It says here to put powder under your breasts to keep from getting a rash," an amused smile found her face. She closed the book and handed it back to me. "Please take care of yourself, Carl," she said. I could feel the genuine tenderness and concern, but something was absent in the reaction I had expected.

"It's about time for me to leave," she said as she gathered her things and stuffed them into a tan canvas bag. Mike's working tonight and I want to see him before he leaves." Michael Parducci was Jill's boyfriend and my best friend from high school. He was a penguin suit-wearing waiter at Montague's in town, an upscale restaurant where the customers tipped well.

"Ok. I'm gonna head on out," I said getting up and moving to the door, "I have homework I don't want to do and Mom wants the grass cut when I get home. Tell Mike I said 'hey' and I'll catch up with y'all sometime this week."

We walked downstairs and out to the circular parking area. We hugged and she walked toward her dorm. I got in my car, cranked the front windows down, then sat with the key in the ignition. Since I was on the road so much, I ate lots of drive-through food, cramming the wrappers and bags behind the front seats. The rear floorboards were usually filled with the remnants of road meals up to the rear seat level, sometimes spilling into the seat, paper wrappers twirling around behind me as I rode with the windows down. Old, stale French fries and burger grease on waxed paper wrappers made the car smell like the kitchen of a fast food restaurant, and not a well-ventilated one. When I went to the gas station, I always filled up at least one trashcan with used paper products bearing the colorful logos of McDonalds, Hardees, Burger King, Taco Bell, and KFC.

Jill had expressed real concern when we were out riding around in that fast food trash-laden car some weeks earlier. Perhaps I had expected her to gush with emotion, to hug me and cry. Perhaps I had expected her to snatch the diabetes book from me and devour it as I had in one sitting. Whatever I had expected or played out in my mind beforehand didn't materialize. I realized other people would care about me, about my health, about my new "condition," but my problem with diabetes was just that – my problem.

I turned the key and cranked the car and drove home very alone.

Chapter 4

"The First Hundred Were Easy," I read off the slide, giving the audience a moment before I pulled them forward. The next slide was the typical "before" pictures every weight loss success story has. The first picture was one taken while camping at Lake Greenwood in October of 2002. In the picture, I still had a ring of hair encircling the sides and back of my head as I was sitting in front of a huge breakfast laid out on a weathered picnic table.

"That can't be me, can it?" I asked pointing at the old photo of me on the screen. "He looks like my older, unhappier uncle." I could almost feel their disbelief in the air. "But that really was me. Look at that HUGE plate of breakfast. Eggs, two kinds of sausage, one of those looks like cheese-stuffed sausage, cheese grits, and I still look like I've just gotten some really bad news." There was laughter from the audience and several people said, "that can't be you." I advanced the frame. The next picture was of me in brick red swim trunks reclining on a pontoon boat bench seat on the lake, one fat arm around a black lab on the seat next to me. I heard gasps as people realized that the four hundred pound person on the screen used to be me. The disbelief in the room was almost tangible.

"And this is me out for a day on the lake," I said, giving everyone a minute to get their minds around the enormous contrast. "Yeah, I actually ate my way to that lard ass lifestyle." I didn't feel the need to be anything but truthful.

I remembered both instances when the pictures were taken. The midsummer day on the lake was so hot that I kept sloshing a towel in the lukewarm lake water and dousing myself with it every few minutes trying to cool off. The camping trip in late October was markedly different in temperature, yet still uncomfortable. The twenty-four foot camper trailer I owned was cramped and I had real issues moving around in it and getting in and out with any sense of grace. Even after jacking the trailer up and blocking it with cement blocks on the concrete pad we camped on, when I moved around inside, the whole camper moved and groaned. Spending time in the "great outdoors" was usually less than enjoyable at my weight.

"I was diagnosed with Type 2 diabetes in 1988. That was nineteen years ago. In 2003, I came to a real decision. I woke up one morning and realized I was killing myself. Slowly, happily, but killing myself with food and television. That morning I cleaned out the fridge of all the foods I loved, that I'd grown up on – cheese and bologna and Duke's mayo and buckets of leftovers. I can't tell you how tough that was. Then moved on to the pantry and tossed out all the chips and dips and snacks I loved so much." I could hear a collective groan from the audience. "My morning fasting blood sugars were over 300. Yeah, 300, when it should have been around 100. I knew that. I worked in a doctor's office where I got that information every day. I couldn't say I didn't know. My A1C was almost 11. Yes, 11, when I knew it should have been under 7 to keep the bad things from happening – retinopathy, neuropathy, kidney damage, hypertension, hypercholesterolemia – yeah, I knew. Add to that no energy, fatigue, sleep apnea. The fat and carbohydrate rich food I loved so much had to go. You don't keep around stuff you know is harmful and you can't stay away from. That afternoon I went to the grocery store and loaded up on good food, real food, unprocessed food that I could eat all I wanted of without worrying about overeating on things that weren't good for me or my blood sugar."

Amy, the nutritionist, was smiling and nodding at me.

"And then," I said, pausing a moment, "I went for a walk. I knew exercise was as important as 'good' foods and that I had to start exercising every day. Walking is the easiest exercise we have. We are bipedal for a reason." I lifted one foot and wiggled it. "Everyone here can get out and walk, even if it's ten or fifteen minutes at a time. You know, when I went on that first walk that day, I was so pumped and ready to go. You know how far I made it?" I paused again. "I made it all the way to my mailbox before getting winded." I let that fact sink in for a few seconds. "I was so incredibly fat, so out of shape, that I couldn't even make it all the way to the end of my street. How incredibly sad is that? But you know what? That first night I made it to the mailbox. The next night I made it to my mailbox and halfway to my neighbor's mailbox. The next night I made it to the neighbor's mailbox. A few nights later, I made it all the way up the hill and to the corner of my street. Now," I stopped and grinned broadly, "now I go to the woods after work and go jogging on the trails out at Harbison Forest." The audience clapped and offered praise.

"But," I began again as the clapping slowed, "I didn't get there in a week. I had to work at it, I had to push myself, I had to get that fitness religion. I had to get out every day and do something, walk as long as I could, and do that plus a little more the next night. I had to want it. I had to give something up to get it. Nothing good in life is free."

I advanced the slide to show a slightly slimmer me, bringing that "before-and-after" sound people make when a person has made a huge, obvious change in their lives.

Chapter 5

Graduation came in November of 1990, a fresh Associate Degree in Business in my hands, after paying the requisite fifty dollar graduation fee and not actually attending the event itself. I left college with no prospects and no plans, a rudderless ship on uncertain seas. The thought of Diabetes scared me for a time, enough to try doing something about it, always short of actual exercise, of course. Exercise meant pain in some fashion, something to be avoided. Potassium became my on-again off-again friend when the leg cramps crept back into my early morning sleep, never failing to relieve the pain within a few days. I cut back on real Cokes and started drinking diet drinks, but they were bland in comparison and I didn't feel the need to cut back enough on what I was eating for it to make any real difference. Without exercise, I was going nowhere. I continued to lose weight but only due to the Diabetic Ketoacidosis resulting from my high blood sugar. When my body had flushed out a few pounds, the bathroom trips became less frequent and my weight dropped to a level where my body tolerated the high blood sugar levels. Since I quit getting the leg cramps and stopped having to plan for bathroom trips, I forgot about Diabetes completely. My weight leveled off somewhere around 300, not that I had an accurate scale or would have bothered to use it had one been available. Besides, I had no way of checking my blood sugar outside of the doctor's office and no intention of making another appointment.

My friend, Darrell Harper, invited me to spend Christmas in Atlanta with him. He lived in an apartment just outside Stone Mountain with a roommate who seemed to be little more than a ghost who left his dishes in the dishwasher. Even though Darrell managed a mall jewelry store from ten in the morning till eleven in the evening seven days a week, he wanted some company. Staying on Darrell's couch afforded me the opportunity to sleep until noon, wander the city in the afternoon, then meet up with him when he got off work around eleven. We passed the nights eating takeout soul food – collard greens, black-eyed peas, dirty rice, fried chicken, or chitlins and maw - and talking about business and sales and advertising.

"Only eat your mamma's chitlins," he told me every time we ordered them, "but you can trust this place," he'd say, a storefront restaurant out of the 70's in a part of town I never knew existed before he took me there to eat.

Darrell tried college, but found success easily in retail, rising quickly from new the person on the sales floor to store manager. When I met him in the summer of 1985, he was rooming with a friend of mine from high school. Somehow, our mismatched backgrounds meshed and we stayed in touch after I moved back home. Darrell seldom said anything about my weight or about how much I ate when we were out together. He might call me "big man" or "big guy," but the names were brotherly, not taunting, never judgmental. We were friends keeping company.

"I'll be getting off early this afternoon," he told me on his way out the morning of Christmas Eve, "let's go eat somewhere decent tonight. My treat."

"Works for me," I replied from the couch. I knew by "decent," he meant expensive and that I couldn't afford it. With no time for dating and little time for spending what he was making, Darrell could easily afford to eat and dress well. Something about his tall, thin carriage – loose, but with the slight attitude of a young man with money earned - fit the tight Jheri curl in with the dark suits, French cuff shirts, and designer shoes. He always dressed as if he was ready for an interview, even when taking garbage to the apartment complex dumpster. The "pre-owned" BMW was a gift to himself for maintaining the highest level of sales in his chain in Atlanta for the year. He let me drive the Beemer to dinner that evening.

"Where are we going?" I asked, adrenaline electric in my arteries as the speedometer glided easily past one hundred, my chubby fingers holding the grey leather-wrapped steering wheel. I could feel myself pressing into the blue leather bucket seat. My little Chevy Spectrum struggled to crawl past eighty.

"Steak and Ale," he replied, pushing Run-D.M.C.'s *Raising Hell* cassette into the stereo and paying little attention to my driving. We both loved speed and the West German auto provided it, carving the cold night air, the dotted center lines stretching into a single white ribbon, pointing us to Christmas Eve dinner.

We strolled into Steak and Ale in Stone Mountain, both of us wearing black suits with trench coats, his dark grey, mine, ubiquitous tan. The restaurant was crowded.

"At least a thirty minute wait tonight. You can wait in the bar," the chipper waitress told us.

Darrell was taller and slid easily onto one of the high barstools, but I had to step on the large brass footrest pipe to get onto the stool next to him. When I put my full weight on my right leg, the thick brass pipe bent to the wood floor.

Darrell wasn't looking at me, but realized something had happened when he turned to see my face, a mixture of fear and embarrassment. He looked down, saw the pipe touching the floor, looked back at me, and started laughing, then caught himself and looked around to see if anyone had noticed, then started giggling. Then he reached over, gave me an arm up, and I settled in next to him, thoroughly abashed. He wouldn't stop giggling. Soon enough I got over my embarrassment and joined him.

Christmas Eve dinner on Darrell's tab was particularly excellent. I ordered a Fred Flintstone sized steak, medium rare, two baked potatoes almost as large as Nerf footballs, billowy peaks of sour cream, and butter, lots of butter.

I didn't need a "to go" plate.

We both spent most of Christmas day napping in front of the television. Darrell was a comfortable friend who accepted me as I was.

*

I started making frequent trips to Atlanta to visit. Darrell gave me a key to his place and I stayed there most often when I was in town. Without college or a job to answer to, I had plenty of time to wander, picking up consulting jobs, usually just enough to keep gas in the car. Home computers at the time were small, black screens with green or amber letters and there were few repair services that would go into someone's home and work on the systems. One of those consulting gigs led me to a startup multimedia company. Harrison Technologies was the idea of an architect who designed expensive houses, the kind with a back porch that led directly onto the golf course green. Being from small town Newberry, I had never seen such huge homes, much less had the opportunity to walk into a place with Italian marble everywhere and bathroom fixtures worth more than my life. The small mansion was new and exciting and I was dazzled.

The two brothers who owned the business scheduled a morning job interview at a McDonalds in Atlanta that I knew well. In my naiveté, I ordered and ate my way through my usual two sausage and egg McMuffins, extra cheese, double order of hash browns, while they explained what the company wanted to do and what they needed to get their plans underway. I was newly twenty-three and they were talking to me about a real job in the big city and I was eating as if lunch were a far-off uncertainty. Moreover, they were paying.

"We need someone who knows something about multimedia technologies, someone who can get the pictures and information from the builders we work with and translate it into a touch-screen kiosk presentation," they told me.

"Sure, I can do that," I said with confidence, "I've been working with optical and scanning technologies and I've been doing lots of desktop to mainframe communications over serial protocols in a hybrid environment of desktop, mini, mainframe, and dumb terminals." I could tell from their faces and the quick glance between them that neither knew what I had just said.

I kept talking.

Working for the brothers at Harrison Technologies was somewhat less than lucrative, but the experience and education were invaluable, far outweighing remuneration. The corporate headquarters for Harrison Technologies was the large house of the brother's parents, a solid structure with lots of hewn wood, handcrafted workmanship throughout. Lunches were often leftovers from the family's previous night's supper. When I left in the late afternoon, almost without exception, I would pull up to the drive through of Hardees, Burger King, Taco Bell, or McDonalds for my post-lunch, pre-dinner snack to tide me over until I could sit down to a full meal at one of my local buffet haunts.

The manager I had worked for as a student at Piedmont Tech, Michael McKinney, had taken a job in Atlanta and had a two bedroom corporate apartment near where I worked. When I applied for the work-study job at Piedmont Tech, I already had something of a reputation with the computer science department's faculty as being a little too knowledgeable for my own good. I hadn't actually done anything to get into trouble, but the possibility seemed to exist, like bringing home a bear cub to raise as a pet. I almost wasn't hired. Mike met with me in his office with the door closed.

"I'm going to give you a chance here," he told me in his National Guard Warrant Officer voice, fluorescent light shining off his balding head and round glasses, "but if I catch you dickin' around with anything you shouldn't," he lowered his voice to menacing, "I'll break your fingers."

I knew Mike was serious and liked him immediately. We became friends, sharing interests in Tolkien and US history. We stayed in touch after college.

When I told him I was coming to work in Atlanta, he invited me to stay with him during the week. Otherwise, I would never have been able to survive on my salary.

Mike lived in Hodges, South Carolina, and had a wife at home working in Greenwood. The job he took in Atlanta was much more lucrative than working for a state college. He usually drove the two hours home on Friday afternoons, returning to Atlanta late Sunday night or going straight to work on Monday morning.

Mike talked about food, his enjoyment of it, his love of cooking, but he never actually seemed to eat. He was a solidly built National Guardsman in his late forties making an effort to stay in shape to meet the Guard's yearly physical requirements. There was a treadmill in his bedroom never used to hang clothes or towels, its motor regularly producing a mechanical drone through the thin sheetrock walls while I kicked back in a recliner, watched television, and shoveled in chips and dip and microwave popcorn, extra salt and butter, until I got too sleepy to get my hand to my mouth.

Home for me was Newberry, three and a half hours from Atlanta; I drove it most weekends to spend time with friends still in college. Logging seven or more hours a week on the road meant I was eating major amounts of fast food in the car. I had my favorite stops: the McDonalds in Newberry, the Burger King an hour away in Greenville, SC, the Captain D's an hour from there in Commerce, GA, the Krystal as I entered Atlanta proper, and several truck stops in between in case I needed Cheetos and a bathroom stop. I knew each of their interstate exit numbers and road names, calculated distance and drive time between their respective off ramps in my head, and knew their drive-thru menus by heart. I developed a system to ensure I lay in enough supplies to last between stops.

One chilly afternoon on my way back to Atlanta, I bought six cheeseburgers and laid them in the sun across the dash to keep them warm as I ate through them. McDonalds had a two-cheeseburger meal and I would get three of them – singles with cheese, onions, pickles, ketchup, and always extra mayo, plus three large fries and three large drinks. I would put two of the drinks in the console cup holders and quickly drink the third so I could set the cup in the front floorboard. Sometimes I would mix it up a bit and get three different soft drinks or three sweet teas. They would give me a small bag filled with ketchup packets. I became quite adept at opening them with my teeth, holding the packet in my right hand, getting fries out of the bag, stuffing them into my mouth, then squeezing ketchup in behind them. The floorboards were littered with white foil packets and bitten-off corners. When I asked for the extra mayonnaise, every single time, whoever was doing the preparation would slop on so much that it leaked out the sides, lubricating the bun such that the meat would slide off in my hand if I didn't hold the burger tightly enough. Warm Duke's mayo would escape the sandwich and wander onto my hand and sometimes down my wrist. Tepid French fries were fabulous with warm mayo, salmonella never a concern.

I stayed in Atlanta for almost two years. Atlanta hosted many cheap restaurants; I slowly worked my way through a serious number of them, mostly buffets. In cold weather, I would wear a heavy coat with lots of pockets and put open zip top bags down in the pockets. Then I would go inside, pay my money, and show the hapless, unsuspecting buffet people what "All You Can Eat" meant to me. When I got home, I would pull out my plunder, plastic bags full of fried chicken, biscuits, hamburger patties, or even chicken potpie if the wait staff was overworked and I was feeling particularly daring that night. The fridge always seemed to hold pilfered leftovers tucked away for later. Often "later" meant simply later that same night.

Gas was still less than a dollar a gallon and my little four cylinder Chevy had a reasonable appetite for fuel. Working at Harrison was good; I enjoyed the people, and living in the Atlanta area. Newberry was a small town with few chain stores. Most everything closed after one on Wednesday afternoons and Belk was the largest department store in town. Atlanta, however, had everything and most of it was open late and weekends, especially the buffets.

Unfortunately, Harrison Technologies ran on a perennially overstretched budget; revenue was an elusive suitor, teasing and tantalizing, yet remaining at arm's length. I didn't see a bright future, and wasn't doing well financially. I went on a few half-hearted interviews in the area, but nothing came of them and I knew I couldn't afford to live in Atlanta if Mike or Darrell's situations changed and I had to find something on my own. I knew it was time to let the big city go and find something near home.

My waistline, in contrast, knew no such budgetary constraints, expanding with each fiscal year, my investments in fast food and buffets showing remarkable returns on investment. The leg cramps came occasionally and I continued taking the potassium supplements. I knew I was gaining weight, but the diabetic symptoms were not as pronounced so I didn't think too much about it. New pants were purchased, worn, outgrown, and replaced. The clerks at the Stone Mountain Big and Tall shop greeted me by name. Their wares were unflattering at best, downright hideous at the lower end of the retail rack. I stuck with solid colors, the darker the better. Basic black always worked. Everything was tight. The last thick, black leather belt I purchased before leaving Atlanta behind in the winter of 1992 was four and a half feet long.

Chapter 6

The slide was still up with a slightly slimmer version of me smiling from the screen. Instead of the big, floppy t-shirts in my "before" pictures, I was wearing shorts and a muscle shirt and had clearly just finished exercising. I wanted the audience to know how quickly little changes in food and activity made a difference in my life.

"In about six weeks of walking and eating better, I was about thirty-five pounds lighter and down two pants sizes. I paid close attention to what I was eating. I carried a food diary with me everywhere and wrote down everything I ate or drank. Food diaries are great. If you use them to write down everything you put in your mouth, I guarantee at the end of the day you will be surprised at how much you are eating, often out of boredom or habit. I kept a faithful diary and got outside to walk every night for at least thirty minutes. I found that I started looking forward to that time out walking. I had time to clear my head and think, time to enjoy my music or an audio book and just be alone with me after a full day of interacting with people. That time became important to me and I looked forward to putting on my walking shoes and headphones and getting out of the house. I tell you, my iPod is the best piece of fitness equipment I ever bought!"

I advanced to a slide titled "Type 2 Diabetes."

"But I didn't stick with it. Things happen. Life happens sometimes. I had home issues that I could do almost nothing about and I turned to food to make me feel better. I lost that religion for a long time. I kept doing some walking and didn't go back to the Chinese buffets. But I didn't keep the fire. I maintained that loss of thirty-five pounds and didn't gain weight, but I didn't keep losing, either. By 2005, I was still having high morning blood sugars and injecting 50 units of Lantus insulin twice a day." I could hear the something from those in the audience who knew about Lantus. Lantus was a twenty-four hour insulin and I had just told them I was injecting huge doses twice a day.

"Yes, 100 units a day and getting nowhere. I knew I was dealing with insulin resistance. My body was still making insulin, but my tissues no longer wanted to use my own insulin and weren't doing a good job using the big doses I was injecting. That's what happens with weight gain, your body develops a resistance to your own insulin. I knew I had to do something. My feet were numb, yet they burned all the time and felt like I had needles poking into them all around. Painful. Nerves are a funny thing. And they don't like too much sugar in your bloodstream. Neither do your retinas. Diabetes is the leading cause of blindness for adults age 20 to 74. High blood sugar increases blood pressure that makes the little blood vessels in your eyes bleed. That bleeding causes damage your retina. That damage, that loss of vision, is permanent. I have little spots in my eyes where I don't see any more." I pointed out across the room. "I have these little grey footballs here and here and here that I simply don't see anything with any more. Every once in a while I'll catch the rear view mirror with just my right eye and the car behind me will vanish. Yeah, that's just a little scary the first time."

I gave them a moment to think about losing their sight.

"And I got up every morning ready to take a nap. I never got enough sleep. Being fat meant my throat was closing up at night and I kept waking up – sleep apnea. I slept eight hours, but felt the next morning like I hadn't slept at all. During the day, I would go to sleep every time I got still. That was bad enough at the office, but waking up as your car is rolling off into the median can be scary and dangerous. Some nights I'm not even sure how I made it home without wrecking the car."

Chapter 7

I had moved home to Newberry some months before and started looking for a full time job. Mom worked most of the time, so we seldom saw each other, almost like having a roommate who paid most of the bills, cleaned up, and left cooked food in the fridge. I was doing a few small consulting jobs, but I needed real work, something that would lead to a career. I wanted to be able to get a place of my own and I didn't have a steady paycheck or benefits.

"What are you doing these days?" Gary asked me on a December Saturday afternoon in a computer parts store in Columbia, South Carolina. I had worked with Gary on a consulting job that paid well, but hadn't talked with him in months. He was one of those people who always had a connection, knew how to play the game of networking, worked a room the way an artist might work in acrylics or watercolor. That kind of social skill eluded me. Gary had a politician quality about him, the ability to move through a room smiling and shaking hands and making small talk, leaving each person with a feeling that they had his undivided attention in that moment. He was a natural salesman and looked the part. I guessed Gary was in his late thirties, but he still had a remnant of "fraternity brother" draped around the edges of his personality.

"Not much," I replied, "just trying to find a steady job. I've been picking up little gigs here and there, but nothing that pays the bills. I'm back home in Newberry."

"You were doing that multimedia job in Atlanta, right?"

"Yeah. Good stuff, but the company wasn't making money."

"Happens. " I could see the spark, "Hey, we've got an imaging group where I'm at now. Systems integrator over on Saint Andrews Road. I know they'd love to get a multimedia developer on staff. He paused, looking at me a little sideways. "You interested?"

I didn't hesitate.

"Yeh, sure. Saint Andrews Road. That's not too far from the house. Maybe thirty or forty minutes if traffic ain't bad,"

"Shorter commute than Atlanta," Gary laughed and pulled a business card from his shirt pocket, flipped it over and wrote on it. "Call me Monday. I'll transfer you."

I took the card, thanked him, and told him I would get in touch with him mid-morning, knowing that computer support issues were always heaviest first thing Monday morning. Gary made good on his promises putting me in touch with the manager of the imaging group, Marlin Alford.

I started work two days later.

*

The Brothers Alford, Marlin and Brad, had a decidedly military bearing. Marlin was an amiable sort, thin and tall with round glasses. He reminded me of Craig Reid of the Proclaimers, and I kept waiting for him to break into a chorus of "I would walk 500 miles." Brad was shorter, more compact, and muscular, like a boxing lightweight. They took turns educating me on what our group had in progress, what we were trying to move toward, and how we planned to accomplish our goals.

When one wasn't speaking, the other was, often picking up in mid-sentence from the other. I was young and excited to work in a much larger company than I was used to, so I soaked in their plans, making them my own, trying to find angles perhaps they had not thought of.

"Let's get lunch," Marlin said to Brad and me just before noon, "I'll drive."

We went to his dark green Eddie Bauer Edition Ford Explorer. They offered me the front seat, so I climbed into the tan leather interior, found the button to move the seat back, then pressed and held it until the seat stopped moving.

"KFC alright?" he asked.

"Fine with me," I said, hearing similar acknowledgement from Brad sitting in the back seat on the driver's side.

I hadn't "done lunch" out of the office often at my previous job. Usually we ate in most days, so leaving the office for lunch daily was new, and I liked the thought of it. Besides, a visit to the Colonel with his delicious eleven secret herbs and spices was always welcome. The Colonel could be counted on to deliver flavor in golden delicious, deep-fried packages, complimented with comfort food side dishes.

I ordered my usual three pieces of extra crispy, double mashed potatoes and gravy, two biscuits, butter, and large sweet tea. When we sat at one of the plastic tables, the brothers each had a chicken sandwich and fries to my large, black Styrofoam plate of the Colonel's fare. Brad was Army Reserve while Marlin was National Guard, so they were accustomed to eating quickly, both finishing in less than five minutes. They sat chatting while

I slowly, methodically ate everything in front of me, leaving no crumbs and refilling my large tea. I refilled my tea once more before we left.

*

On my way out of the office at the end of the day Friday, Gary called to me from the bottom of the stairs. "How's the first week, Superstar? I don't remember us ever hiring anyone on the spot."

I gave him a big grin and a chubby thumbs-up. "Good enough. I think it's gonna work out fine."

"Good deal. You get along with the Alford Boys?"

"Yeah, seem like nice guys. They're both still back there working," I said, nodding over my shoulder.

"They do that. Both of them live about two minutes from here. First in, last out."

"Well, it's taking forty minutes to get here, so I'm a bit farther out. I need to get on up the road," I said, thinking that my favorite reruns would be on about the time I rolled into the yard. Dinner was a ritualistic affair on the couch with Kirk, Spock, McCoy, and the weekly Disposable Redshirt Crewmember who died in the first ninety seconds of most episodes. "Tomorrow," I said, "and, thanks again. I really appreciate the referral and the reference." My appreciation was genuine.

"Not at all. Now you owe me," he said, winking and turning back down the stairs and out of sight. The company execs, sales staff, and labs were downstairs, and Gary managed the state sales contracts. He meant that I owed him and would call in the marker when he needed it.

Most every afternoon, I would leave the office, get on the highway, then exit at the next off-ramp to go to a favorite convenience store. The store sold a huge grey plastic mug for a couple of dollars that I could refill daily at the soda machine for a dollar. I always bought a large bag of Cheetos to go with it. Usually I got the crunchy kind, but I gave almost equal attention to the puffed. If by some happy circumstance the special issue waffle Cheetos were on the shelf, I would purchase several bags of the large, crunchy, square goodness to savor in the car and in front of the television. I would eat the entire bag of whichever one left the store with me along with the extra large soda on the way home. My fingers were adept at finding every single orange crumb in the bag, before gnawing the salty, cheesy residue off each chubby digit in turn.

I began spending time on the road traveling for the company, eating in the car. The job began as tech service calls locally before growing into overnight stays out of town. We got a large installation job in Hickory, NC, about two hours from the office, and I began spending four or five days a week on site. Living on an expense account was a new experience. I took my queues from my boss, tracking mileage, staying in reasonable hotels, and eating quite well on the company's check. We never spent extravagantly, but I made sure to get at least three full meals and snacks every day along with the requisite receipts, never cheating the system, just enjoying the latitude of it. Working as a road engineer could be a tough life, but the late nights, eating from vending machines, and adolescent humor made it feel similar to college in many ways. One of our employees sent to work for a partner on the West Coast borrowed one of their company vans one night, got drunk, and wrecked it. There was very much a fraternity atmosphere and serious lack of professionalism in the ranks.

"We need a Lotus Notes administrator," Marlin said to me one day. The new Notes email and combined database system was replacing the old email system. Somewhere in the plans, the imaging group took on responsibility for its enterprise-wide rollout and administration. "We think you'd be a good admin. You want the job?" he asked.

"Will I come in off the road?"

"For the most part, yes. We'll still send you out now and again when it's something just you handle." There were several skill sets in the organization I was supposed to be the authority on, though I never understood why or how that happened. More than once I had become the expert on a particular piece of software while at a customer's site with the customer looking over my shoulder. Adrenaline motivated. Being out on the road had its moments, but I was ready to settle for a while. Perhaps Marlin noticed I was getting a little restless. The company had an odd notion of loyalty. Management expected employees to be staunchly loyal, they just didn't bother to reciprocate. The environment felt something like working as a bartender – if I didn't want the job, there was always someone else who did for the same money or cheaper. Several of the pre-sales engineers were friends of friends hired from local sports bars. The quality of their job quotes reflected it. The time in my life, the work, the experience was good training, though, and I knew it.

"Sure. Love to," I said.

"Great. I'll get you admin rights and whatever you need to get started. Figure out what that is, and make a list," he said, then turned for his office.

Lotus Notes Administrator. Can't be a bad thing on the resume.

With that, I became the email administrator for the entire multi-state organization, and began sitting in a chair sometimes for eight hours or more a day, snacks filling my desk drawers, Cheetos at the ready, like puffy orange cartridges in a gun belt. When I did travel to regional offices, I stayed in reasonable hotels. The local office's employees took the opportunity to dine on my expense account under the guise of business, so we ate exceedingly well – steak, seafood, numerous buffets, and rivers of beer. After traveling to each of the satellite offices, I realized one afternoon that I was easily the largest employee on the payroll, but no one ever said anything directly to me or made me feel like an outsider. I practiced the art of self-deprecating humor and was always good for a job or a good-natured jab. I wasn't happy, but I was working and seemed to fit into the mix.

*

Sometime in late summer, I woke up one Saturday morning with a large knot in my right inner thigh. Touching the spot was painful. I thought perhaps it was a bruise, though I couldn't remember doing anything to get it. The pain got worse, the knot growing wider and becoming harder that day. By Monday morning, the hardness had expanded to about the size of my palm and felt something like a golf ball lodged under the skin. This wasn't the first time I had something well up under the skin only to go away in a few days, but this hurt more than it had before and I was starting to get concerned.

As dedicated as I was, I never called in sick or took vacation time. I had never called in sick to any job and didn't even know what the protocol was for telling my employer I didn't feel up to coming in. I had bought into the "you're too important to be off" propaganda management used to motivate a workforce of underpaid youngsters. The rhetoric worked. My leg, however, was increasingly painful, throbbing with my heartbeat, and I wasn't going much farther than the bathroom, the kitchen, and bed.

Just after eight, I called the office and got Marlin and told him I had done something to my leg and didn't feel like I could get out of the house.

"Take care of it and let me know how you are," he said and that was it. I had called in sick.

I stayed in my king size waterbed with the television on, alternating between sleeping and flipping between channels of inane daytime programming. The pain grew worse and I kept running my hand over the spot keeping track of growth throughout the day.

Tuesday morning around five am, the pain woke me. My thigh was rigid and burning. The knot in my leg had grown and felt as if it was going to explode, and I knew I had to do something to try to alleviate the pain. The hardness had moved in a thickening line toward my groin and toward my knee. The hard area was expanding outward as well. I was alone in the house and knew I didn't want to wind up in the hospital, didn't want to have to call and ambulance for something as benign as a big bump on my thigh that had swollen up and hurt. I had health insurance but had never used it and knew nothing about how it worked and I knew I didn't want to try to pay for a visit to the ER or an overnight hospital stay.

I got out of bed and got the Gerber pocket knife that was always in my right pants pocket, then limped into the bathroom and laid a white towel on the carpeted floor. I kept the knife exceptionally sharp. I felt around and located what I thought was the center and softest spot on the growing knot then used the sharp knife point to open up a soft spot in the knot in my inner thigh. Something physically popped, like snapping a large piece of bubble wrap, but didn't hurt. The amount of blood was amazing, frightening, soaking the towel and the carpet underneath. I stood there with my right foot on the tub watching and waiting for what felt like an hour as the wound drained.

When the bleeding slowed enough that direct pressure from a light blue hand towel stopped it, I picked up the soaked towel from the floor, tossed it into the tub, took a dry towel, and pressed it into the carpet. Then I went back to the bed and lay down, the hand towel pressed between my thighs. I was spent.

The wound continued to drain a slick white and yellow fluid. I went through a stack of towels, but it continued to drain unabated as my leg grew even larger. I realized it was a serious infection and that I needed antibiotics to keep it from getting worse, so I called my mother at work to tell her my leg was worse and that I needed medication. She was staying with an Alzheimer's patient so she hadn't been home in days. I left out the story of draining a pint of blood onto her carpet.

"I'll come home for a while after lunch. You need to go ahead and call down to the doctor's office and see if they'll call something in for you," she told me.

I hung up with Mom and found the thin Newberry and Prosperity phone book, looked up the number, and called. The receptionist told me she'd take the message and have the nurse call me, so I lay back in bed and waited.

The ringing woke me. I explained my situation to the nurse.

"Sounds like you have a bad infection. You're Diabetic, correct?"

I realized who the nurse was.

"Yes," I stumbled.

"Well, with your being Diabetic, any infection could become serious. Even fatal. Any problems in your lower extremities should be addressed immediately. You need to get in here now so you can be looked at."

"I can't drive like this and my mother can't leave work long enough for that." I summoned up something pitiful, "Is there any way you can call in some antibiotics for this?"

There was silence for a few seconds. I didn't want to go to the doctor even if I had transportation, but I didn't want her to pick that up over the phone.

"We'll call in something for you, but no pain meds, and you need to get in here as soon as you can. Alright?" She wasn't asking.

"Yes, ma'am, thank you." She asked for some basic information and what pharmacy I used, then ended the conversation. I called Mom and asked her to pick up the medication on her way home.

*

My mother was appalled when she got home and walked into my bathroom to find bloody towels in the tub, but she took it with her accustomed stoicism. She brought me the antibiotics and helped me get laundry started and the bedclothes changed before she went back to work. I took the pills, washed them down with copious quantities of orange juice, and went back to bed.

The rest of the week was painful, but I responded to the meds quickly. Tylenol helped ease the pain. I called Marlin daily to tell him I was still sick, but didn't elaborate and he didn't ask. I was able to return to work on Monday, though I still had some soreness in my right leg, limped slightly, and had to sit on a pillow all day. Only a close coworker, Elizabeth, even bothered to ask why I had been out and if I was doing ok. I told her the truth and she offered sympathy but I realized then that even though I was surrounded by dozens of people working near me, I was alone.

*

The day after Thanksgiving, I was out shopping with my mother in Columbia. We pulled into a car dealership to window show. The Lincoln dealership had a 1993 Executive Series Town Car off lease with a few thousand miles on it that I took for a test drive and fell in love with. I didn't need a car or a car payment, but for the first time in my life, I actually fit in a passenger car without feeling stuffed into the driver's seat. The large leather bench seats were amazingly comfortable, the armrests barely pressing against my sides. The salesman didn't have to talk me into the purchase, I had to have it. I went inside, signed the loan paperwork, and, at age 26, drove home in an opal grey town car whose typical first time buyer was age 62.

*

Monday morning I eased the big Lincoln into the drive thru at McDonalds to order breakfast, the first good fast food I had enjoyed in a week. I ordered two combo meals and ate breakfast off my new leather dash, stuffing spent wrappers back into the paper bag instead of tossing the trash behind the front seat. When I got to the office, I parked my new grey land yacht out front. Although I wanted to email everyone in the Columbia office, I didn't tell anyone I had bought a new car. I kept the news to myself all day letting the kept knowledge warm me.

The following morning I enjoyed my commute as never before. I got to the office, parked, went in, and tried to log in. My account seemed to be locked. I tried to log in a few more times before wandering over to the server room. I could see our network administrator through the glass doors as he sat at his workstation.

"Hey, what's up?" I asked as I entered, realizing something was wrong when he looked up from his keyboard.

"I'm sorry, man. You need to go see Tom," he said. I could see the pain in his look. "I can't tell you anything," he said.

I knew whatever was happening wasn't good news. I also knew that he was an administrator and just did what he was told, so I walked past him and through the opposite door into the management area.

The short walk to the business manager's office was a gauntlet of eyes over the cubicle farm, the eyes of people who knew something I didn't, who wanted to see what was happening, but remain detached, voyeurs. When I got to Tom's door, Marlin was in one of two chairs opposite the desk, the other chair empty and waiting for me.

There was the typical business rhetoric of "downsizing" and "cost cutting measures" and "strategic plans," but the message was that I was out of a job and that I could look for my final paycheck in the mail. I left Tom's office with copies of several job listings in town that I was either not qualified for or not interested in.

That chair saw several employees of the Columbia office before noon. The company wanted to reduce the bottom line in preparation for a buyout. I had never been escorted off the premises of a job site, but, as an administrator, I understood that in their eyes I had suddenly become potentially dangerous. The moment was surreal, happening to someone else in a movie. At the same time, I was on fire with adrenaline, my mind working too slowly to appreciate fully what was happening. Too quickly, my personal items were dumped in a box and I was sitting jobless and alone in my new Executive Series Lincoln Town Car.

Chapter 8

The slide was titled "Progress This Far."

"I've come a long way since 2003. I've lost over 120lbs. My A1c has dropped from almost an 11 to a 5.5 – dead perfect. You couldn't ask for a better A1c. I'm off the insulin and all the anti-diabetic medications." The room erupted in applause. I knew that almost every person in the room was at least on the oral medications if not injecting insulin daily. Once on the meds, diabetics rarely got off of them. No one got off insulin injections, it was just unheard of. With insulin being an anabolic steroid, most people gained more weight, continuing the cycle.

"That's right, I take no meds not because I have to. I still think, since I was diabetic for nineteen years and have done all kinds of damage to my body, that I need to be taking Metformin and Lipitor and an aspirin daily, but I don't have to take anything to keep my blood sugars under control. Anything, that is, but the prescription of eating right and exercising. The copays are less expensive. The important thing is that the neuropathy is gone."

I knew that once nerves were damaged, they seldom got better. Mine had. More applause.

"I feel both feet just fine, passed a monofilament test with no problems, and they no longer hurt or burn at night. My cholesterol dropped from 255 to 144. Yes, I'm still on low dose statins, but I just think that's a good idea. My vision prescription has stabilized. My prescription used to change throughout the day with the sugar-induced changes in my blood pressure. I've gone from XXXXL shirts to XL and Large shirts. And I think I have a good forty pounds to go to reach my goals. I would really like to weigh 220."

The title of the next slide—"The First 100 Were Easy"— brought laughter into the room.

"No, really," I began, "the first 100 were pretty easy once I caught the fitness religion and made it a part of my life. That's the thing, weight loss and blood sugar control, the two are inseparable, are a lifestyle change. You have to want it badly enough to make changes to your life. Little changes make big differences over time. Humans do things either to avoid pain or to gain pleasure. We have a real social problem of wanting everything now. We just can't put off pleasure for later; we can't do something that is a little painful now to get a greater pleasure reward a week, a month, a year, ten years into the future."

I advanced the slide - "The World is Against You" - as I talked on.

"Obesity and Type 2 Diabetes are Social Diseases." I let that sit in the air a moment before going on.

"Our Western Lifestyle of convenience is slowly killing us. There is a McDonalds, Burger King, Hardees, and Starbucks on every corner of our civilized life. There are processed, fat-laden, sugar-filled foods within minutes of most anywhere. Add to that overflowing grocery shelves, convenience foods, cheap buffets, and 'Biggie Size' everything, and it's no wonder we're a fat nation growing even fatter. It's no wonder that diabetes is epidemic. There are something like 20 million diabetics in the US and the numbers are growing at an amazing rate. This is caused almost exclusively by obesity. As a nation, we are digging our own graves with a spoon. And mass marketing drives us toward brand loyalty. We eat at McDonalds because there is a sale this week or a game piece we can collect in a contest to win more food. Add to that what I call the Playstation and Plasma TV effect. We come home from work or school and plop down in front of the TV to watch 100 channels or play video games for hours instead of getting outside and doing something physical."

I tried to engage the audience directly for a moment. "Do you remember what happened when we came home from school?" I heard murmuring in the back of the room. "Yeh, we were told to get outside until we were called in for dinner. We played in the neighborhood, rode our bikes, built forts, whatever, we did something physical. I was the fattest kid in school, but I did at least get out every day and ride my bike or walk to the 7-11. I was still in better shape than many of the kids today, it was high school when I slowed down and started getting serious about packing on the pounds. Now we don't let our children go out after school because we're afraid something will happen to them, so we park them in front of the electronic babysitter and shove food in front of them and that's what they do for the afternoon instead of getting exercise."

I could hear acknowledgment from the room.

"And I love a salty, crunchy snack, now. Cheetos – oh, Lord – I call it the Orange Cocaine."

I waited for the laughter the line always invoked.

"Oh, yeah, the Orange Cocaine. I love it. Crunchy. Puffed. I don't care. Oh, I loved those waffle ones they would come out with around the holidays. And you would be eating along on these things and get this big blob of nothing but salty cheese – OH, LORD!"

Laughter and recognition swept toward me.

"How I did love me some Cheetos, still do. They are tough to pass up. I can't bring the things into the house. And I could easily eat a bag on the way home – not the tiny bag, I'm talking about the big bag at the gas station."

My next slide was a huge picture of a bag of Cheetos front and back with the nutrition box showing on the left side.

"Did you know that one big bag of Cheetos contains 1600 calories – 1600! That's almost an entire day of calories! And 100 grams of fat! 100! And 150 grams of carbs! And 2900 grams of sodium! All that is right there on the wrapper we never read, that Nutrition Facts box that is required on all packaged food. One bag of Cheetos is enough to clear out your entire day of calories, fat, carbs, and sodium in one cheese and salt-fueled sitting! That's just wrong. And I would sometimes eat two or three bags in a day. A day! And that's just snacks, not the buffets I would do all the time. It's no wonder I weighed 400 pounds. Taking in that kind of calories a day with no exercise will pack it on quick."

"Most people never take the time to read that nutrition facts box and I never did before I started really paying attention to what I was shoving in my mouth while I was driving or sitting on the couch watching TV. I certainly didn't care back then so long as what I was eating tasted good and there was plenty of it. When I did flip the bag over and read what the manufacturer considered a single serving and what I considered a single serving, then did the math, I was shocked. I couldn't eat eight or ten Cheetos and stop. Who can? I knew then I had to quit them like quitting any bad habit – put them down and walk away."

Chapter 9

I drove straight from my place of recent employment to the unemployment office in Newberry. The new Lincoln looked out of place in the lot. I had passed by the building in downtown Newberry often enough, but never been inside, never wanted to know what was behind the dirty glass doors. But I knew that unless I wanted to sell the new car, I had to go inside and beg for a weekly check from the government. Not having a job was so foreign to me. I wasn't supposed to be out of work involuntarily; I was supposed to be in demand.

I wondered if they would ask me about any recent large purchases.

The unemployment office was everything I expected, and less. The room was half full with the sort of people I'd imagined would be there, the chronically unemployed by choice, the day laborers, and a couple of guys who smelled of formaldehyde and looked as if they simply had nowhere else to be at the moment, perhaps former mad scientists past their prime. They accented well the gloss tan-on-concrete-block décor.

The requisite paperwork took nearly an hour to complete. I sat at a chipped white Formica table and waited my turn. The woman who finally took my application wore a purple wool jacket with a gold floral print that reminded me of my grandmother's love seat. The jacket was roughly the same size as the loveseat, too, I considered as she smoked and coughed the whole time I sat in front of her in a folding metal chair, breathing in what felt like second-hand failure.

"Since you're what we label as *professional*," she said, putting an annoying emphasis on "professional," "you can take your job form around to local employers and get them to sign off on it." She paused to drag on her cigarette. "Or you can send us back the form filled out each week with copies of at least three letters you send to potential employers with your *resume*," again putting a little English on "resume" as she stared at me through the blue haze, ash falling from her left hand onto her purple jacket.

"I would prefer to send in copies of letters with my form," I said.

She paused. "I thought you would," she said dismissively as she began moving papers on her desk, stapling them together, then handing me ten or twelve pages. "We'll process your claim and you'll hear from us in a week or so." Her body language indicated clearly we were done.

"So I won't get a check for a week?" I asked, having had no experience with the unemployment system.

"We have to process the claim first and get information back from your previous employer," she explained in the same condescending voice she had undoubtedly used with thousands of newly unemployed before me. "If it's a valid claim and your previous employer doesn't contest it, you start collecting a check the second week." Something in me waited to hear her say "dismissed," but she just put me out of her mind and went back to moving and sorting papers on her desk. I showed myself out the dirty glass doors into the warming November sun.

My watch and stomach both indicated it was lunchtime, the watch being the lesser accurate. With the hint of honest green still in my wallet, I drove to Burger King, ordered two Whopper with cheese meals at the drive thru, parked in the adjacent parking lot, and sat eating in the car with the windows down while listening to the radio. I might as well enjoy a last meal out before the money was gone, I reasoned.

Unemployed.

There was such a stigma to the word. My mother had worked since she could walk, going straight to the cotton fields in the late 1920's. She was a workaholic in the sense that she never sat still when there was something that "needed doing." In my mother's world, there were always things that needed doing. I hesitated to even think how she would react when I told her. Telling her about my new employment status was not something I looked forward to. Being laid off, fired, would add to the litany of disappointments I had handed her over the years. We would survive. We always did.

My biggest concern was how much money I would get monthly, assuming my claim was valid and the company didn't fight it. The mental tally of monthly expenses grew. I was sitting in the largest grey leather upholstered expense on the list. Good jobs were hard to find, and I didn't want to start working for minimum wage somewhere while trying to find something comparable to the job I'd lost. Not many employers would want to be little more than a bridge between jobs, allowing me to cut work to go to an interview or use the office phone to make calls to HR managers and follow up on job leads in the paper. Besides, I had worked at a McDonalds one summer during college and hated it. I cleaned the McBathrooms, mopped the McFloors, and picked up McTrash in the McParking lot. The bullfrog green 100% polyester shirt and pants uniform was insanely hot, didn't fit well, itched, and trapped sweat like a plastic garbage bag. Even when washed daily, there was always a McAroma permeating the clothes. I collected two McChecks before dropping off the company-owned Kermit suit, vowing never to work in fast food again. I looked down at the empty greasy bags in the front floorboard and wondered if the Mighty King of Burgers required polyester uniforms of his subjects before I quickly shook the thought of going in applying. I finished my second cardboard pocket of fries and drove home.

Later that evening, Mom took the news stoically. She always surprised me by not reacting to big news the way I expected. Usually things I considered insignificant set fire to her rockets, likely her method of coping with things outside her sphere of influence. Her history was compiled of circumstances and decisions she had little control over, little power to change. I seldom made it any easier.

The first days of my liberation from the responsibilities of a job were like a long weekend with no impending Monday morning. I had never taken vacation in the year I was with the company, so I enjoyed my new freedom. I began staying up late, sleeping long past sunrise, and catching a nap on the couch in the afternoon.

Some of my still-employed ex-coworkers started calling me. Internal memos and resumes appeared in my email. The layoffs were a surprise to everyone; the transient nature of their job scared them. People who didn't know me when I was packing my personal effects started acting like best friends. Most asked me to keep them in mind when I landed a new job. The corporate grapevine I wasn't privy to while an insider longingly extended itself to me on the outside. There were whispers on the wind that the company was up for sale and the layoffs were a means of cutting costs, showing a better bottom line without increased revenue. If that were the case, I was probably better off looking for something than waiting out the unknown; an academic question at best. I was without employment and real friends and needed to move on with my life.

*

The unemployment claim went through without incident. My former employer listed our collective terminations as "layoff," qualifying us to collect an unemployment check. An envelope with The South Carolina Employment Security Commission at the top of the return address was in my mailbox after my second week out of work. Since Newberry was a small town, those at the post office who sorted the mail, and long time mailman, Dale, knew I was "on the dole." I waited for him to put my mail in the box and walk up the block before I went out to get it. Our bank didn't have a drive-thru window or I would have used it instead of making my weekly Deposit of Shame in person, the pretty blonde teller always asking how my mother was. The monthly total the state bestowed was well below what I was used to, but, living at home, I was able to get by without giving up snacks or television, the cornerstones of existence.

*

"I've got a lead for you, Buddy," my ex-coworker and friend, Daron, told me in a phone call just after New Year's. "Meet me for lunch tomorrow. I can't talk now."

Daron always had a gift for putting buyer and seller together. He was the image of a young Andy Garcia, exuding charm and charisma, backed by a solid understanding of voice and data communications. He had the most well appointed office, a large closet under the stairs leading into the drab computer lab. From Daron I learned of Eileen Gray, Le Corbusier, Mies van der Rohe, Marcel Breuer, and George Nelson - modern furniture designers. He had a Wassily chair and two Barcelona chairs wedged into his small under-stair hideaway. I couldn't wedge my big butt into most of his furniture.

We met at a sandwich shop in Columbia. I ordered a huge Ruben with an extra pickle, chips, and a large drink.

"The university has issues with their new Citrix server. Their IT guys bought the software from us and installed it, and now they don't know what to do with it. They're talking about using it for dial-up access for the enterprise if they can get it configured and running right," Daron told me as I tore into the delicious sandwich, the warm Thousand Island dressing running out onto my hands. He picked at his chicken sandwich. Daron lived on hard candy and four hours sleep a night.

We were the only two Citrix Certified engineers in the state at the time, and I was the only OS/2 Certified Trainer in South Carolina. The position was a solid fit and we both knew it. "I talked with the tech guy over there yesterday," he continued, "and they're looking for a network guy. They'd really like to find someone to manage the Citrix box. I told him I knew who they wanted and I'd ask you to get in touch. So, you're interested, right?"

"Of course" I need a job bad. This paid vacation has been fun, but I'm not making money, and I don't have insurance."

He gave me contact information, and I called when I got home.

"Can you come in tomorrow?"

I panicked. My suits didn't fit. I hadn't needed one for over a year, and had long since outgrown what hung in my closet.

"I'm actually busy the next couple of days," I lied, "do you have something later in the week?"

I held my breath. I could hear paper moving.

"Sure. How about Friday at ten?"

"Yes, that's perfect. I'm free all day Friday." After I hung up, I found my Columbia phone book and flipped to clothing – Big and Tall.

I grew up wearing a Sears line of clothing for fat kids called "Husky," and I hated having the label on the back of my pants. I wanted to wear the same label clothes as the other kids in school, but I never could as the token fat kid in class. When I went looking for a new suit, the salesman gave me the adult name for the size I wore. I had graduated from "husky" to "portly." After trying on many pairs of slacks, each about a foot too long, and suit jackets with sleeves almost to my knees, I settled on a flat black suit with tiny streaks of color woven into it. I didn't like the suit nearly as much as I liked the end of having to shop and try on clothes. The image looking back at me from the mirror as the salesman marked me up with white chalk was not that of a man happy with his purchase. The last suit I had worn was several sizes smaller.

The salesman found a long leather belt and "Big Man" white shirt, and promised me the alterations would be done in time. He then went to the counter and started adding up my bill. I wasn't prepared for the total. Big & Tall meant out of the ordinary, expensive. The extra few inches over what was an "off-the-rack" item commanded a premium price, four times what a similar one was on the rack at my local K-Mart. The same applied to the white dress shirt, the slick white version with too much polyester in it. The base price for the suit was not unbearable, but the alterations cost more than the suit. I felt like I was buying a base model car and adding leather and chrome wheel covers. My credit card would take a bit more punishment, but I had no choice, I needed interview clothes and I hoped the suit would buy me the job. So I laid the grey PNC MasterCard on the counter, signed the receipt, and walked out with my new belt and shirt.

On Friday morning, I walked back into the store and tried everything on. Realizing I didn't have a tie, I bought an extra long, equally expensive tie the salesman suggested, then drove to the university for the interview. Although the suit technically fit me, nothing was comfortable. Even in January with the windows down I was sweating, and not from nervousness. I didn't usually get nervous when my technical knowledge and skill sets were the question, I was just hot.

The networking department supervisor met me as I came off the fourth floor elevator. We chatted for a minute in the hallway before he led me to the office of the Director of Computer Services. I hadn't expected to be interviewed by the department director, but I was glad the interview was starting out at the level. Perhaps they were serious. Perhaps they were desperate. The director had a quiet, imposing air about him, but my technical portfolio was complete, and I had no problems answering their questions. The interview went quickly, too quickly.

"So, how much do you need?" the director asked me. When I said the number, I knew instantly they were relieved, leaving me with the feeling I could have asked for a higher salary. The networking supervisor took me out to show me around the office.

"We haven't actually posted the job, you understand, so we can't actually offer you anything today. But, um," he paused, "what kind of working area would you need?"

*

The interview felt like it went well, even promising, so I felt there was cause for celebration. I knew most of the good buffets in the Columbia area and there was a country cooking buffet I had not been to in some time, so I went there for a late lunch, careful not to get anything on my new, expensive, extra long tie.

The hiring process took just over a week to complete. My first day at the university was January 24, 1994. My new boss, the networking department supervisor, wanted me to attend an IT conference and had instructed me to go straight to Owens Field in downtown Columbia to fly on the university's airplane to Washington, DC, for the day. I had flown in small planes before, barely wedging into the tiny seats. Fortunately, there were bench seats on the university plane, though I faced backward and there was no snack cart. I had to wait two hours for a standup lunch at a counter at the hotel convention center.

The conference was a good introduction back into the working world and an opportunity to mingle with new coworkers. We got along well and walked the convention floor for hours. I was winded, my feet hurt, and I was delighted to get back to the plane to fly back to Columbia. On the way home that evening from the airfield, I stopped at the convenience store I frequented and loaded up on drinks and snacks.

*

I settled comfortably into my new state job, which was much easier and less stressful than the private sector. The hours were set, coffee and smoke breaks often, chatting over cubicles plentiful, and the lunch hour observed religiously. At five fifteen, the office was deserted. One of our interns, a young, compact ex-marine named Patrick, and I started working closely together on projects and became friends. We started having lunch together and found we shared a love for cheap Chinese cuisine, the kind of small buffets most often found in strip mall storefronts. We decided to start with the first listing for Chinese food in the yellow pages, and tried to eat our way through all the Chinese buffets in Columbia.

We made it better than halfway.

Chapter 10

I clicked off the nutritional label slide to a picture of a table loaded with all manner of fast food from doughnuts to chili cheese fries.

"And that's the thing," I said pointing to the photo, "you have to have food. Some studies suggest that losing weight and keeping it off long term may be harder than kicking heroin. I've said this before and I've had mixed reactions from recovering alcoholics, but I just believe that the guy with an alcohol problem can choose to avoid the bar, or choose not to bring home that twelve pack of beer. The lack of alcohol may be painful, but it won't kill him. You can't choose not to eat. We are biomechanical machines engineered to take in food and turn it into energy and store what we don't use. As a society, we are geared toward instant gratification – especially here in America. We want it NOW! McDonalds and Starbucks and Dunkin' Donuts are there to fill that need, that wanting it now, instant gratification. And often the cheapest food is the worst for you. People have done studies on this. The segment of society that is living on welfare buys food that's welfare-approved. That list reads like a how-to for packing on weight, developing hypertension, and promoting diabetes. I'm not kidding!"

Heads nodded in agreement.

"Look at what our American lifestyle is doing in other countries. In every country where we set up our fast food restaurants, something like a generation later, the obesity rate, the heart disease rate, the diabetes rate changes; it begins to match the American rates – which are beyond epidemic. Numerous studies show that the American lifestyle is downright lethal over the long term."

"It's a daily battle," I said as I advanced to the next slide, "a battle we wage every day with every forkful, every cardio session, every walk, every weightlifting session, every breakfast, lunch, dinner, and snack. We have to take this seriously with every piece of food we eat, what we drink, every time we talk ourselves out of going for a walk because it's cold outside or we've had a rough day or don't have time. I know, I talk myself out of exercise all the time. It's easy. I can rationalize away most anything. But the thing is, I'm just shortchanging myself when I do that, when I skip an hour at the gym on a Tuesday afternoon. The reality is, that if I'm feeling rundown or just feeling down, ten minutes into my workout, I'm going to feel great. When I leave the gym, I'm going to be in much better shape all around – physically and mentally – than when I went in. That's the secret. That's the payoff. And I understand how tough that is."

I paused again.

"I know how tough it is to go to the gym, especially the first time. As a university employee, I have free access to the school's gym. I remember going to the university gym for the first time. I changed into a pair of black XXXL shorts and a big, floppy black t-shirt at the office and drove to the gym and parked out front. I sat there in the car for maybe thirty minutes before I got up enough courage to go in. I was waddling into a gym where extremely fit college students were. When I did get out of the car, I walked up and held the door for a girl coming out. I swear she had just stepped off the cover of *Surfer Magazine* – the girl was just perfect – great tan, tight outfit, towel wrapped around her waist, long, black hair still wet from the pool, wraparound sunglasses – and she looked right through me. I wasn't even there. As huge as I was, she had no problem completely ignoring me. I can't even begin to tell you how much that hurt. That was hard to deal with."

I could see nods and acknowledgement around the room.

"Fortunately that didn't stop me. But it certainly could have. The invisibility of fat people just amazes me. So many times I have passed women on the street or in the grocery store and I could just tell they made an effort to keep from making eye contact. There were so many times in my life when I was the largest person in the room, but people didn't seem to see me. So many times I was just ignored, overlooked. But even knowing that people ignored me to my face, I was still hypersensitive about walking into a gym with all those young kids. That was tough. But I did it. I went in and worked out for the first time since high school. When I say worked out, I mean I tried a few weight machines, not knowing what I was doing, got worn out quickly, and left. But the important part is that I was back the next day and the next and the day after that. I began to enjoy it. I got used to the soreness. I picked up a book on weightlifting and learned something about muscle groups and what exercises work what muscles and how to alternate workout days. No, I didn't get it right the first few weeks, but I was doing something. That's the key – do something. And I was walking every night, too. Aerobic exercise – walking – is the number one thing you can do to manage your weight and blood sugar. I walked.

And I tracked my numbers. Keeping up with your data is extremely important. Food diaries are a great way to start. You also want to weigh yourself every morning. I work in a family medicine practice and we have these hyper-accurate, Satanic scales in the office."

Several people chuckled.

"My doctor told me I should weigh every morning about the same time and naked, which was fine with me. Unfortunately, a few of the nurses complained."

Chapter 11

Later that year, I was sent across town to work on an email server for the School of Medicine. I quickly learned that there was an opening for an Information Technology Manager in the Family Medicine Department. I met Dr. Lindsie Cone for lunch at The Shrimper for the formal interview. After I was hired, the everything-is-battered-and-deep-fried-and-sided-with-hush-puppies restaurant became one of our weekly lunch destinations.

*

When I started working at the Med School, I was dating a tiny redhead in Dayton, Ohio, roughly ten hours away. We had met on the phone a couple of month earlier. She was working phone sales at a cable supply house I purchased from regularly. Almost every time I called in an order, I got her and I just loved her voice and her laugh. Soon, if she didn't answer, I asked to be transferred and waited for her to finish another call. After a time, I called her simply to talk. When I got up the nerve to ask her for her home phone number, she surprised me by actually giving it to me, not something I was used to having women do. I called her that night long distance, and we talked for at least an hour about everything in our lives. That was before generous cell phone and unlimited long distance plans. I did not know it then, but she was as lonely as I was. She was almost eleven years older and quite cute in a long cotton, peach skirt and bobbed red hair that changed hue weekly from the manufacturer's dark brown, never one to make up her mind and keep it made.

When she lost her job, I would send her gas money and she would make regular road trips to South Carolina and spend a week or two with me. My mother was not pleased. We did, however, have a lot of laughs and ate well and enjoyed the newness of it all. We got engaged early into the long distance relationship that lasted from February through November. Her life was as well rooted in Ohio as mine was in the South, but there were deeper issues. One of the last things she said to me almost pleading was, "You won't change for me. You won't lose weight. You don't really love me."

She was right, of course. My weight was remaining steady, but I wasn't even trying to address it. We went out to eat often, ate anything we wanted, and I never exercised. I was just enjoying being with a woman who wanted to be with me.

Then she left.

*

New coworkers meant new lunchtime haunts – fried seafood, BBQ, country buffets and, of course, Chinese buffets. My assistant and boss tried to make it out of the office for lunch together five days a week, succeeding most of the time. My boss, Dr. Lindsie Cone, also my primary care physician lectured me occasionally on how much I was eating and how my weight was affecting my life that diabetes would eventually lead to all sorts of bad things. Although I heard him, Lindsie finally resigned himself to the fact that I never listened or cared enough to do anything about my health.

"Diabetes is the number one cause of blindness in South Carolina," Lindsie said as he watched me shove in sesame chicken and wash it down with glass after glass of cold sweet tea, "and the leading cause of kidney failure. You don't want to go blind and live on dialysis. Do you know how many of my patients had their legs amputated as a direct result of uncontrolled diabetes? I see it every single day in patient care, noncompliant patients who won't watch their diet and won't exercise and won't take their meds."

I knew those statistics, certainly, but somehow they didn't apply to me. I was in my twenties, and felt relatively indestructible. All my medical problems were decidedly minor. Besides, diabetes didn't hurt. I had been diabetic for years and I didn't feel like anything permanent had been damaged.

My weight continued to increase. My hips and knees and ankles cracked most of the time when I got up and down. I got winded walking across the parking lot. Business attire for me grew to be black jeans and black t-shirts, if not slimming, then functional. I tried to dress merely to meet the thresholds of temperature and decency. I neither knew nor cared anything for fashion and I only bought clothes when my old ones no longer fit. I hated having to go to the Big and Fat store for pants that cost twice as much as their normal sized cousins at K-Mart plus the cost of alterations. I hated those stores and hated having to shop in them. All of the pants I bought were at least a foot too long as if only giants had waists that large and their taste in fabric leaned heavily on 100% polyester. The company obviously had a policy against hiring fat people in executive management or they wouldn't have hung their hideous wares out for sale.

I was well dressed in a suit and tie, however, the day I walked into a local electronics supply house to purchase parts for something broken at the office. The woman behind the counter had waited on me before and I had always been impressed with her knowledge of the store's inventory and pricing. Slightly shorter than me and of average build, she had a new, unflattering perm, gold-rimmed glasses, and laughed often while juggling a counter full of customers, all male. When it came my turn, I handed her a part we needed. With database efficiency, she rattled off the part number, how many they had in stock, and how much it cost. I was impressed and took note of the distinct absence of a ring on her left hand. When she came back from the storeroom with my parts, I handed her my card and said, "if you're free some Saturday evening, I do great dinner and a movie," paid for the parts, and walked as confidently out of the store as I could manage. She paged me that evening. We talked every night. I made her laugh a lot. I enjoyed connecting with a woman again who actually liked me.

She moved in with me some months later and we took up housekeeping. She'd been renting a house with a older male roommate and she seemed eager to exit that arrangement. When her dog died, we found a replacement puppy at the local pound, a black lab / cocker spaniel mix I named Ruff, a prophetic name. On Valentine's Day in 1999, I gave her an engagement ring and she gave me a Springfield 1911A1 .45 automatic pistol. At the time, I figured any woman who would give a gun as a Valentine's present was a keeper. Eight months later, on the deck of the cruise ship carrying us on our Caribbean honeymoon the morning after our marriage, I knew it wasn't going to work.

Chapter 12

I wanted the audience to understand that managing their weight, managing their blood sugar levels, was a daily struggle.

"Studies show that people who weigh every day do better over time than weighing once a week. It has something to do with daily feedback. You want to keep track of your weight every day, your blood sugar readings every day, and your exercise. I got a cheap pedometer, a little gadget that looks like a pager that counts your steps as you walk. I got one of those and wore it every day. Health experts tell us we should all be walking at least 10,000 steps a day. I know that sounds like a lot, but that's really only around five miles a day and an easy number if you are just the least bit active. To keep track of my walking, I wrote down the number of steps I took every day and tried to log at least 10,000 steps every day. The pedometer I bought counted steps as well as miles. So, every night when I got ready to go for a walk, I checked it before and after and wrote down the mileage just from walking. The first year, I walked over 250 miles. I know when you say 250 miles it sounds like Mount Everest to anyone who hasn't been active. The key, of course, is that some nights I walked a whole mile and some nights I walked three miles. Each night built on the next and added up over 365 days."

I advanced to the next slide, "The Glycemic Index." I raised my hand and asked, "Who has heard of the Glycemic Index?" Hands went up around the room.

"The Glycemic Index tells you something important about the foods you eat in relation to your blood sugar. Anyone like Chinese food?" I saw some smiling faces nodding back at me. "Who doesn't? Oh, yeah, I do love me a Chinese buffet. We used to hit the buffets almost every day for lunch and I couldn't eat sensibly. I had to get my money's worth as well as two or three skinny people near me money's worth, too. I loaded up my plate and went back for more. But what do you always say after eating having Chinese food?"

Several people gave a similar answer, "You're hungry an hour later."

"Why is that? Have you ever checked your blood sugar after a big Chinese food fest? I did. My blood sugar levels bolted up after a big Chinese buffet lunch. Then I was hungry later in the day. Now, mind you, I still felt full, but I was ready to eat on top of that. Why is that? The reason is found in the Glycemic Index."

"Chinese food," I continued, "is heavy in carbohydrates – rice and vegetables. Carbohydrates, especially simple carbs like sugar, soft drinks, candy, white rice, boost your blood sugar quickly. They have a low Glycemic Index (GI) number. The lower the GI number, the more quickly that food has an effect on your blood sugar. White rice has a low number, lower than brown or wild rice. So, what happens when you eat and your blood sugar goes up? Your body pushes insulin into your bloodstream to bring the level down to something normal. Insulin brings down your blood sugar level. What happens when your blood sugar gets low? You get hungry. So you eat again. The cycle begins again. With simple carbs, you eat, you get full, then you get hungry again not long after, then you eat again. The Glycemic Index shows how easily you can get trapped in that cycle, staying hungry all the time."

I saw recognition in many faces and people leaning into each other talking low.

"I quit drinking regular soda; regular soda is packed with high fructose corn syrup. Regular soda is little more than liquid candy. I drink diet sodas and cut back on how many of those I drink daily. Studies have shown green tea is so much better for us. I drink it often with lemon and Splenda. I use the yellow stuff, the blue stuff is tolerable, but that pink stuff is the work of the Devil! My mother used to make iced tea with saccharin and I never got used to it."

A lady with bright white hair and the greenest suit, shoes, and handbag I had ever seen put her hand up and asked without preamble, "So, how do we break that cycle?"

I turned and gave her my full attention. "The easiest way is to cut back on simple carbohydrates. Consider the white foods – white rice, white bread, grits, white potatoes – all have lower Glycemic Index numbers which mean they have a quick and mesurable impact on your blood sugar levels. The simple advice I have for these foods is 'White Ain't Right.' If you avoid these white, high index foods whenever possible and eat them only in moderation, in small amounts, your blood sugar levels and hunger will be much more even throughout the day – which is what we want to see. Substitute brown or wild rice for white. Swap whole wheat brown bread for white bread. Try a sweet potato with Splenda brown sugar and low fat butter. I hate sweet potatoes myself any way you cook them, but they are much better for you than regular potatoes. And I sure do love me some mashed potatoes and gravy, now. I was raised up Southern, so in my house, we even put sausage gravy on the sausage."

Chapter 13

I knew I snored, had always snored, would actually wake myself up sometimes in the recliner snoring. That didn't bother me so much, but I hated being tired all the time.

Monday mornings were always tough. My alarm clock was the kind with the largest red numbers possible because of my bad vision, and the alarm was the loudest the Federal government allowed in a consumer product because I could easily sleep through it, incorporating the shrill beeping into my dream. I always woke up tired and ready for a nap. Rolling out in the morning wasn't getting easier.

"You scared me again last night," my wife would tell me, "you would stop breathing for a while, then gasp, then let out a huge snore." I always shrugged it off, but I knew I couldn't continue night after night sleeping and not getting rest.

"What you're describing is called sleep apnea," Dr. Cone told me one afternoon when I was complaining about being sleepy and telling him the wife said I stopped breathing during the night. "You weigh so much that your throat is closing up at night and you stop breathing, then gasp for air. That keeps you from getting a good night's sleep. That also puts stress on your heart. Sleep apnea increases your risk of high blood pressure and heart disease. If you weren't already diabetic, sleep apnea increases your risk of becoming diabetic and increases your insulin resistance. You really need to go for a sleep study."

Naturally, I never did.

Between the sleep apnea and getting up to pee every hour on the hour through the night, I wasn't getting solid, restful sleep. My daily commute was an hour each way and I would go to sleep in the car driving down the highway. Many mornings I would not remember most of the trip into the office. "My car knows the way to work," I joked, but driving sleep-deprived was dangerous. I dealt with the added stress by eating.

My feet added to the nighttime distraction. My toes and the sides of both feet were numb, but when I went to bed, they burned and it felt like tiny needles were sticking into them from all sides. Pain medication did nothing for me and the jars of creams and lotions I tried were a waste of money. Some nights were tolerable, but often it felt like my numb, tingling feet were suspended over a campfire, not quite hot enough to catch flame or char flesh, but hot enough to burn.

In the middle of one of her serial unemployment cycles, my wife began sleeping during the day and spending most nights playing internet games and chatting on the laptop dusk till dawn, so many nights I lay in bed alone so tired I could barely stay awake, but too uncomfortable to drift off into sleep. The widening distance and resentment in the marriage didn't help settle my mind at night, either.

Chapter 14

The slide with the food-laden table was still up and I knew I had at least one nutritionist in the audience who was available to the participants.

"Ok, we stop drinking regular soda, we start eating low carb, low fat, low sodium, and low calorie. I have a nutritionist in my office who gave me that same advice. I told her that the only thing that was low carb, low fat, low sodium, low everything was dirt. She told me to mix it with spring water and make a nice mud pie. Great."

I moved on to the next slide, "Eating Right."

"Seriously, you want to limit the amount of food you eat in a day – calories – but you also want to put those calories to work for you. Consider, we are biomechanical machines engineered to take in food and turn it into energy. Simple carbs like refined sugar is very easy for our bodies to process. The majority of metabolism – and we'll cover metabolism here shortly – the majority of calories burned in metabolism are during digestion. So, don't you want your body to have a tougher time processing food into energy? Sure. That means you are using up more calories to process the food."

"Ok, let's walk through this slowly. Say you eat one of those popular 100 calorie packs of crackers. For the sake of simple math, and realize these numbers are not accurate, they are for us to talk this through, but let's assume your body expends 10 calories to digest that amount of food and to turn it into energy your body can use. That means you have 90 calories left for your body to do something with. Let's also assume you eat that sitting at your desk in your office and you are doing very little physically to need those calories. Say you use another 10 calories as you move your mouse around looking on eBay instead of working. That means you have 80 calories from that 100 calories pack of crackers that is leftover. What happens to them? Yeah, those 80 calories finds their way to your thighs. And once those calories get stored there, it is tough to get them to come back out for energy."

"I'm simplifying this like crazy, but you get the idea. Assume you eat a 100 calorie piece of lean, grilled chicken breast instead of crackers. Chicken, meat, are what?"

Several answers came from around the room. I picked out the most obvious.

"Lean chicken breast is protein. Sure, there's some fat, but let's assume that it's pure, grilled, protein goodness, complete with grill marks, ok? You eat that piece of chicken and your body starts working on it. Here we have a change, though. Where simple and complex carbohydrates have a relatively small 'caloric cost' associated with digestion, protein 'costs' more for your body to digest. So, where those crackers cost 10 calories to digest, let's say the increased cost for this chicken is 45 calories. What's happened here? Well, we had 90 calories left over when the crackers were digested, but the chicken has only 55 calories left over after digestion. So, we are looking at a difference of 35 calories here. If you still only use 10 calories surfing the net at your desk, then only 45 calories – half the cracker number – finds its way to your thighs. And the other part is that chicken, meat, and protein have a much higher Glycemic Index. Protein does very little to boost your blood sugar, so you get full and stay full much longer on meat than you do on carbohydrates. You won't want to eat again as soon, so you eat less throughout the day."

"I know this is a lot to take in, sort of like trying to get a drink from a fire hose. But this is basic biochemistry and we all need to be aware of how food affects our blood sugar levels when we eat certain foods.

Chapter 15

"Your blood sugar readings are just too high, Carl. You're going to have to go on insulin." I was sitting on Cone's dark blue couch in his small office listening to him and feeling the room constrict even more. I had been a diabetic for more than a dozen years and getting nowhere in managing my weight or, in turn, the disease. A rift opened inside me and I was in two places, the person sitting on the couch listening to a medical diagnoses, and an observer in the room watching the scene of doctor and patient, transmitter and recipient of bad news. The patient received the information, but was not processing the ramifications of what was said. Perhaps it was shock or nearness to the situation, but the patient side of me remained calm, detached. The observer, however, had done enough reading to know what "going on insulin" meant: injection, needles, pain. If the patient wasn't frightened, the observer was.

That evening I was home alone with our two dogs as I often was. My wife was never home, always out with friends or on an extended trip to visit family, so I was used to having the house to myself.

"I'm going to visit with my aunt in Memphis," my wife announced one evening as we were eating dinner on wooden TV trays in the living room during Jeopardy. The wife had filled the house that evening with the delightful smell of Southern fried chicken and surrounded the golden-brown, crispy bird on my plate with a small mountain of mashed potatoes and a lazy river of brown gravy made from the chicken bits left in the pan. A can of biscuits and a huge glass of sweet tea rounded out dinner nicely. She had once worked in a truck stop as a short order cook and could turn out a solid comfort food when she had a mind to, which was less and less often.

"How long will you be gone?" I asked around my fork.

"Oh, I don't know, maybe a month or two. She's having surgery and I'm going to look after her for a while. She doesn't have anyone else. And I need a vacation."

She always told me what she was going to do rather than ask my opinion. Since I was the one working in the family and she was usually off with her friends, I wondered why she needed a vacation.

"I'm going to need a bus ticket for next Saturday," she said, and the conversation ended.

We were well acquainted with Greyhound, having left the driving to them on many of her trips – Memphis, Tennessee, or Evansville, Indiana, or Point Clear, Alabama. The routine was always the same, I paid for the ticket, gave her some pocket money, and dropped her off at the local Greyhound station, then awaited her return. Sometimes she would be gone for a few weeks, sometimes months. Her trip to Memphis in 2003 lasted almost a year.

*

I had purchased and taken home an insulin pen, a metal and blue plastic tube about the size of a rich man's cigar, pre-filled with a mixture of fast and slow acting insulin with a place to screw on small, single use needles. I already had a box of alcohol pads from the office.

"These are the smallest gauge needles made. They shouldn't hurt at all," the pharmacist told me. I didn't believe her. Needles were needles, sharp sections of metal designed to penetrate flesh, not unlike a knife, only smaller. Needles were invaders on domestic soil, something to be avoided and guarded against.

"When you were small," my mother had told me often when I was younger, "when you had to have your shots to start school, it took the doctor and three nurses to hold you down."

My thoughts on needles had changed little in the ensuing years. I couldn't remember the last time I'd had an injection. Checking my blood sugar with a steel lancet was a daily painful necessity, but jabbing a piece of sharp surgical steel into my own flesh to deliver medication into fat and muscle was quite another undertaking entirely. Not only was there the aspect of self-mutilation that touched my primal nature, but the was the visualization of the entire clinical process: pushing in a needle, avoiding whatever anatomical things might lurk in my arm, pressing down on a plunger to deliver the liquid, waiting for all the medication to come surging out of the hollow steel, then pulling the metal from my flesh. The lancet hurt for a moment and a drop of blood appeared at the injury site. I was used to that, knew the process and what to expect. I was not a trained phlebotomist with experience with needles and medication delivery. I thought I could probably inject a patient successfully, but being the patient and delivering the injection myself was just overwhelming.

I checked my blood sugar with a meter I kept on the back of the toilet. The small device required an expensive, single-use test strip that wicked blood down into the machine to analyze. While I was supposed to be testing first thing in the morning and throughout the day, I usually only performed the routine once a day. A type 1 diabetic or seriously type 2 diabetic without insurance who tested their blood sugar levels regularly as recommended could easily spent $150 or more a month just in test strips. Even with quality insurance and free boxes of strips from the meter reps coming through the office, I still wasn't following doctor's orders. I hated the routine and didn't like what the meter told me day after day, that I was weak and couldn't control something as seemingly simple as blood sugar. My approach was avoidance. If I didn't get the morning readings every day or several times throughout the day, I didn't have to think about it. No sense hurting myself physically only to hurt myself mentally.

Most mornings, though, I did check and would pull one of the strips from the container and slide it into the top of the meter, take out the plastic lancet "shooter," put in a new lancet, pull back on the arming device, put the tip on the shooter on the side of third finger of my right hand, press the trigger, and jump. The tiny steel stiletto pierced a hole in my flesh quickly and efficiently. Then I would squeeze the finger to get a large drop of deep cherry to touch to the test strip. The meter sucked the liquid in, thought about it for a minute, then displayed my numbers on an LCD screen. My numbers were always high. Too many mornings my blood sugar and weight came rather close to matching, somewhere around 375.

That evening after dinner and well into prime time viewing, I took the prefilled insulin pen from the refrigerator where I had stored it next to the sticks of Blue Bonnet margarine in the door, then went to the living room and flopped down in the couch in front of the television. The coffee table was a low, rough-cut, heavy wood table I had bought along with matching end tables for $90 in Atlanta third or fourth hand at a used furniture store. Across the table was a white towel with the cold insulin pen, a box of needles, and a box of alcohol wipes on it.

"Most diabetics give themselves injections in the fatty part of their stomach," the pharmacist had told me. Although I had plenty of "fatty parts" to choose from, the thought of plunging a sharp object into my abdomen was beyond my ability. I decided I would try the most common place I had received shots before and, being right handed, selected my upper left arm somewhere between where I guessed my bicep and tricep touched under a protective layer of fat, more educated guess than anatomical certainty.

Setting up the insulin pen was simple enough even without the huge foldout instruction page in tiny writing. The pharmacist told me to begin with 20 units and monitor my blood sugar readings and adjust the dosage as necessary. I took a disposable needle cartridge from the box, unwrapped it, and screwed it onto the end of the pen. When I uncapped it, there was a gleaming inch or so of sharpened surgical steel protruding from the white plastic mounting. I couldn't even imagine how much it was going to hurt to stab myself. The needle penetration was only the first step.

The pen had a clear window on each side so the glass insulin cartridge would be clearly visible. The glass was a little foggy from condensation. I wiped the glass so I could see the medicine in the cylinder. Insulin was a clear liquid with what looked like a little seminal fluid in it. There was a tiny glass ball in the cylinder.

"You'll want to rock the pen side to side so that you mix up the insulin," the pharmacist told me. "Never shake it, use the little ball in there and rock the pen back and forth in your hand like this." She demonstrated the proper way to prepare the shot. "It will take a couple of minutes to mix it thoroughly right out of the fridge, but be patient. Remember, don't shake it." I wondered why the pharmacist instead of my doctor was demonstrating the proper administration of insulin.

That evening I sat on the couch slowly rocking the pen and watching the little glass bead travel back and forth through the liquid as it grew cloudier, like semen, I thought with an accompanying spinal shiver. Once the medicine looked completely mixed, I looked even more intently at it wondering if it had warmed up enough or too much, and if temperature would affect how much it hurt in my arm. I wondered if the liquid would go right in or make a bubble. I was required to have a yearly PPD test at the office to see if I had been exposed to tuberculosis, and that always made a little bubble under the skin that itched like a huge mosquito bite. I hated those. The mosquitoes in my back yard were rabid enough; sometimes I could swear they traveled in patrol squadrons loudly humming Wagner's *Ride of the Valkyries*.

I stared at the gleaming needle and the tiny hole in the angled tip, something reminiscent of nightmares. One television show ended and another began, the inane chatter of loud commercials lost in the background as I focused on the singular moment, the threshold from being normal and not having to have insulin to being dependent on the anabolic steroid for the rest of my life -- to keep from going blind, to avoid the amputation of the lower extremities, impotence, kidney failure, and a host of other diabetic complications. I knew the disease, knew the symptoms, and knew the outcomes. I saw patients wheeled into our practice with one or both leg stubs wrapped in cream colored stretchy socks.

"You know as much about diabetes as I do," my doctor told me more than once. I knew I didn't want to become another patient in a wheelchair.

I took the pen in my right hand and slowly put the tip of the needle against my skin. I felt the pressure of the metal tip. I reached out my index finger and gave the top of the pen a tap. The sharp metal didn't pierce my skin like I had expected it to. I tapped again and the skin held, making a small indentation under the needle. I could feel the tip pressing against me, unpleasant, but it didn't actually hurt. I tapped again a little harder and metal disappeared into flesh. While I felt it, the pain wasn't what I had expected. There was an initial sting, but once that was over, I had a foreign object embedded in my body, but there wasn't real discomfort. I moved my thumb to the plunger and pressed. The pen made a clicking noise as the plunger slowly came down, as medication was forced from the pen, through the needle, and into my body. Ten clicks and twenty units of 70/30 insulin had been transferred from the glass container into me.

I slowly slid the needle from my arm and a single drop of crimson blood leaked out of the broken skin. I set the pen on the table, tore open an alcohol pad, and wiped the area thoroughly. The sharp odor of alcohol reminded me I had just performed a medical procedure, one of many I would endure, having joined the populace of the insulin dependent.

Chapter 16

"Oh, here we are at metabolism," I said with some anticipation in my voice. The slide had a black background with a large bonfire in the middle of it, a graphic I found somewhere on the net when I was putting the presentation together.

"How many people here have built a campfire or a bonfire or watched someone do it?" Most of the room, as I knew, had had that experience. The fire metaphor was steeped in history and mythology.

"How many times have you said or heard someone say that they had a slow metabolism and that's why the weight just packs on? Or their skinny neighbor or coworker had a high metabolism? What are we talking about here, this metabolism thing? Well, you don't have to be a physiologist to work through this one. Metabolism, simply, is how many calories your body uses throughout the day to maintain itself. This is easy math. If you have a slower metabolism from living a slower lifestyle, and you eat more calories a day than your body uses to maintain itself, you are going to gain weight."

I pointed to the campfire graphic on the screen. "So you want to go out and build this big bonfire? What do you do? How do you get it going? You get all your big logs together that you want to burn and stack them up and just set fire to them and you get this big, roaring fire that burns all night, right?"

I looked around the room to see some confusion and shaking of heads.

"No, that doesn't work, does it? How do you start even the largest of forest fires? The first thing you do is get together a few small twigs, maybe some shredded newspaper or cotton balls soaked in petroleum jelly, and you light that with a match and blow on it and start this little fire, right? That smokes along a little bit, catches a small flame, and you tend it along. You start adding more fuel to the fire and it gets a little larger. Then you put on some bigger sticks, then branches, then eventually, when you have worked on this fire for a while, you can put in a larger piece of wood. That's how it works, doesn't it?" I asked and saw agreement.

"Then what?" I continued. "You've got the size fire you wanted so you can just go sit down and watch it burn the rest of the night, right?" More dissension in the room. "No, doesn't work like that, does it? You have to tend the fire, right? You let it burn down a little, you poke the coals with a stick, you add a little more fuel. You can't leave that fire for very long without it dying back down, so you work at it, you tend it, the entire time you want flames and heat. And you don't just dump all your big logs on at one time and expect the fire to consume it all at an even rate, do you? No. So, the question is, if a fire can't handle all that fuel at one time, why do we sit down to three big meals a day and expect our bodies to use that fuel over a twenty-four hour period?"

I let that question sit in the air for a good twenty seconds.

"Exactly. We have been taught that breakfast, lunch, and dinner are how we are supposed to go through our days. The reality is that the 'three squares a day' mentality came about as a convenience; scheduled feedings lends itself well to an industrialized community. We get up, eat a small breakfast, get out the door, break at noon by the office clock, work all afternoon, get a dinner, then park in front of the television for prime time viewing. This has nothing to do with the natural working of our bodies. It's wrong!"

I saw nods in the front row.

"What we should be doing is grazing throughout the day. This plays out not only for our metabolisms, but for leveling off blood sugar levels. What happens when you pile on the food three times a day? Your blood sugar spikes three times a day. We don't want that. The well-controlled Diabetic, the patient that has the least symptoms and the best clinical outcomes over time, is the patient who keeps their blood sugar on a nice, even curve throughout the day. The patient who loses the most weight and keeps it off is the person who spreads their eating out over the day instead of funneling it in three times a day."

"Anyone heard of *Body for Life* by Bill Phillips?" A few people raised their hands. "Bill Phillips owned a bodybuilding supplement company some years ago and ran a nationwide contest. He put up an Italian sports car, his blood-red Lamborghini Diablo, and a spokesperson contract to the person who showed the most improvement following his twelve week fitness plan. Something like 54,000 people entered the contest. What's important about this for us is that in the data-gathering process, they found that regardless of age, fitness level, weight, and so forth, the single variable that tied all of the success stories together was spreading out meals throughout the day. Those were the people who showed the most improvement. So, what am I saying here? How do you go home and use this? Simple. Take what you are eating right now – let's call it an 1800 calorie diet because I can do the math on this one – six times three is eighteen. Take the 1800 calories of food you are eating right now and simply split that up into six 300 calorie meals. Go heavy on the protein and eat about 300 calories six times a day beginning right after you get up in the morning. What does that do for you? Simple. We want to bump our metabolism up so that we get the ongoing calorie-burning effects from things like digestion. So, we keep putting food – fuel – on the metabolism fire in small amounts to keep the furnace stoked at a reasonable, constant level. This also helps keep our blood sugar level on a constant line throughout the day because we aren't pouring in food we really don't need. If we are eating high protein foods in reasonable quantities, there isn't going to be a big insulin release so we aren't going to get hungry for no good reason. If we aren't hungry, we aren't going to eat food we don't need in between. You may still want to eat for some psychological reason, but the physical signs of hunger won't be present."

"And, always, eat when you are hungry. I tell people all the time that if I get hungry, it means I didn't plan well. So I keep snacks around my life that are low in sugar so I won't get a blood sugar bump between meals. You want to pre-position food around your life so you won't give into a quick bag of Cheetos or a burger off the dollar menu. That's too easy. And what you will also find is that once you are exercising regularly, your appetite will drop off. When I was working out the hardest, the toughest part of my fitness plan was remembering to eat. I know how that sounds, but it's the truth."

"What about eating before bedtime?" I asked. The murmuring in the room had a distinctly negative tone.

"OK, so we're told not to eat before bedtime, right? Let's look at that. If you go to get at eleven and get up at seven, that's eight hours you are going without eating. That's why they call it 'breakfast – breaking the fast' – it's like going to work in the morning with out eating and working all day without eating. That's not good. We want to go to bed with food in our stomach. Remember what we just talked about, about metabolism being inextricably tied to digestion? Well, when we stop eating at seven or eight in the evening then don't get breakfast until seven in the morning or maybe not even until lunchtime the next day, that whole digestion process has mostly nothing to do until you eat again. So we want to keep food in there, right? Sure. When professional bodybuilders are training for competition, many of them eat before bed and set their alarms for the middle of the night to get up and eat another small, protein-filled meal. Seriously! They do that to keep the anabolic process going. They don't want their bodies to have the opportunity to tear down lean body mass overnight which is what happens when you fast for any length of time. That's not anabolic, that's catabolic, and we want to keep that from happening. Lean body mass – muscle – is our friend."

"So, what do we want to eat just before bed? Maybe a big bowl of vanilla ice cream?"

I heard the negative reaction.

"No, of course not. Ice cream is loaded with fat and simple carbohydrates. No, we want to get some protein in there that stays in the system for a while. Since I love low fat cottage cheese, that was a natural for me. Low fat cottage cheese is a fantastic food staple. I know many people don't like it, but I'm lucky enough to be able to all but live off the stuff. A cup or so of 2% cottage cheese right before bed is enough to keep my insides working until breakfast. I suppose a turkey sandwich or wrap would work well, too. You have nutritionists here at your service," I pointed at Amy, "and I'm sure they can help you find something that you like that serves the same purpose. Use your resources."

Chapter 17

I was at my favorite Chinese buffet, the one with the four long lines of heated, Plexiglas-hooded aluminum tables steaming with all manner of foods I loved, and the discolored metal Mongolian grill at the end. Traditional Cantonese string music played from ebony, wall-mounted speakers. I recognized the place as the restaurant I frequented so often the wait staff had long since stopped asking me where I wanted to sit and what I wanted to drink. There were weeks when I had eaten there eight or more times, lunch and dinner, under the huge pictures of blue and white waterfalls and Hong Kong's waterfront after dark hanging on the walls over the booths. Sesame and ginger clung to the air as one of the cooks banged wooden sticks on the grill, sautéing mushrooms, shrimp, and mixed vegetables together with teriyaki sauce, the delightful, campfire-like crackling sound of frying loud in my ears.

The tiny waitress dressed like a soft ninja took me to a freshly-wiped table, faint streaks still apparent on the cheap, tan laminate surface. I dropped my keys and went straight for the stack of hot, still-damp white plates; I took one off the top stack and immediately began loading it with pork fried rice. General Tso appeared to be in fine form, so I piled on his spicy, dark-sauced chicken, crispy Crab Rangoon, and golden, deep fried chicken, then went back to my table and dropped heavily into the black vinyl-topped chair to dig into my plunder. A dark amber plastic glass of sweet tea and a paper napkin-wrapped, dishwasher-battered fork and butter knife were waiting for me - tools of the trade.

I started shoveling in the Americanized, MSG-laden version of Chinese food as I always did, eating away at my first plate while thinking about what I was going to get on my next trip to the steaming trough; teaching the hapless, unsuspecting buffet people that I took "All You Can Eat" as a personal challenge, an affront to my eating prowess. When I went to buffets, I meant to get my money's worth and, perhaps, the money's worth of one or two skinny people sitting near me, more a financial than culinary decision. The dull, stainless steel fork kept moving between plate and mouth, but something odd was happening, the plate didn't empty.

I continued to eat.

When I took food from the piled plate before me, the voided space seemed to fill back in. I took larger forkfuls. The amount of food never changed. The tea glass I drank from never held less. I looked around the room, but everyone else appeared to be enjoying their meal, eating, then returning to the metal tables for more or sitting in conversation. Whatever was wrong must have been just with me.

I continued to eat.

Even more food began replacing what I had taken from the plate. After a couple of minutes, the pile of rice and the General's chicken had grown to five or six inches high and began spilling over the edge and onto the table. Crab Rangoons crawled from under the rice, off the plate, and onto the table. I couldn't shovel and chew and swallow fast enough to keep up. The pile of Chinese food continued to grow until the plate was covered completely; rice and chicken cascading off the sides making a large, rising ring in front of me. Tea began rolling over the top of the plastic tumbler, onto the table, spilling onto the floor.

I continued to eat.

The food grew to over a foot high in front of me, a river of tea spilling onto the floor, soaking my right sneaker. The other patrons did not seem to notice what was happening with me. I kept shoveling food into my mouth, chewing as fast as I could, swallowing, then going in for more, the mass of rice and chicken continuing to grow in front of me. After what felt like fifteen minutes, the original plate had grown to a mountain covering half the table and beginning to roll off into the floor. I pushed back from the table in disbelief. I realized that I was not full; I was actually still hungry, but frustrated and confused.

The dark-haired, dark-eyed ninja girl walked over to me.

"Oh kay? You need more tea?" she asked.

"I, uh," I started, wondering why she didn't see what was happening. "I seem to be having a little problem here."

"No problem," she said, "you eat yourself to death now. You need plate?" she asked, waiting for my response, smiling serenely.

The room suddenly grew freezer cold. The table legs buckled as it slammed to the floor under the weight of the food that had grown into a small mountain in front of me. Rice and chicken and tea splattered all over me as Crab Rangoons scuttled away to hide under bench seats.

Then I was awake. My heart was hammering in my chest. Cold sweat soaked my hair and the pillow. I gasped for breath. There wasn't enough air in the room. After a few seconds, I realized I was at home in bed and not at the Chinese restaurant.

Then came the fear.

The dream, the tiny Asian waitress, had been so vivid, so real, tactile in every way down to the spicy crunch of the greasy chicken in my mouth. My stomach even felt full as my mind tried to explain what I was feeling.

Eating myself to death.

Something deep inside my subconscious knew it was true, what the waitress said, I was eating myself to death. At nearly four hundred pounds, I was huge and miserable and suffering. The weight had been part of me, was me, for so long. The pounds had moved into my life quietly an ounce at a time, a teaspoonful at a time. Food was comfort, a friend always there when I needed it, a lover with an agenda – to keep me all to itself. Fat surrounded me, imprisoned me, and I knew it, had always known it. Ready access to all the food I wanted and sixty channels of premium cable television conspired openly to keep me insulated, isolated from the world, from possibility and potential, future and success. Certainly I was married and held down a good job, but there was no joy in my life, no real hope for tomorrow beyond planning the next night's television viewing and requisite snacks, which buffet to choose the next day – Chinese or Southern Cooking. My life revolved around eating, the next meal, one more trip to the buffet tables, catching every episode of my favorite Prime Time programs. When I sat down to dinner, I spent the whole time planning what I would have for breakfast and lunch and dinner the next day, never enjoying the constant assembly line of food I was cramming in my mouth. Pleasure was about having, not enjoying, quantity versus quality.

I was ashamed to think my life was nothing more than Cheetos and Star Trek, nothing more than food and entertainment, nothing more than immediate pleasure at the expense of future. The worst part, what stabbed at me the deepest, was that I knew better. I knew how to eat right and exercise and check my blood sugar levels daily, I had every medical resource necessary for good health available to me free of charge where I worked, but I didn't take advantage of it. How many times had I gone to lunch at a Chinese buffet with my doctor and, under his disapproving, disappointed glare, eaten four or five plates of food along with four or five glasses of sweet tea? How many times had he bitched at me out of love or frustration to get my eating under control and to get some exercise? How many times had he counseled me about the dangers and eventualities of being morbidly obese and diabetic? How many times had I simply ignored him, brushed him off, continued to stuff Cheetos in my face, gnawing the salty, cheesy residue off my fingertips after meticulously cleaning out the bag?

I was thoroughly ashamed of myself. Thirty-six years old and my life was at a standstill, parked in front of the buffet, tanning in the glow of the big screen television. The adrenaline-charged thumping of my heart eased some, leaving me with a genuine pain, the hard soreness of loss. My eyes shut tight against the tears finding their way in hot streams down each side of my face, falling in splatters on the pillowcase.

You are eating yourself to death. I heard in the voices of the little Asian waitress and my mother at the same time.

Mom was always feeding me while telling me at the same time that I needed to "get some of that blubber off," maternally loving, yet insensitive. I knew I was hearing the truth. I was killing myself slowly with a fork and a television remote. That guy who weighed over a thousand pounds and had to have a hole cut in the side of his house to get him out to load him on a flatbed trailer to get to the hospital once weighed what I did. He didn't expect to weigh a thousand pounds, didn't get up one morning and decide to be as big as a pickup truck. He got there, though, and did it the same way, eating like a recently freed prisoner of war, and lying around like an invalid. I could weigh a thousand pounds, be imprisoned in my own house and body, make the local news, a mountain of lard hauled away on a flatbed trailer like a wrecked truck.

The tears came more easily. I began sobbing. I had always been fat. I had always been "big boned." I had always been the "jolly fat guy," good for a joke and a laugh, usually the self-deprecating kind, and I hated it. I hated seeing the fat guy in the mirror every day, the one with no self-discipline, no self-control. I hated that bastard, wanted him dead. He wasn't me.

Wanted him dead.

A small, quiet voice deep inside finally spoke up.

That's it, isn't it?

I was doing everything I could to murder the fat guy I hated, murder him carefully and systematically. The poor idiot thought I was being good to him all along, feeding him lots of food, keeping him from the pain of exercise, entertaining him. All the while, I was slowly poisoning his system, burying him in layers of fat put on one delicious ounce at a time. The plan had taken decades, but he was morbidly obese, had few friends, had horrible blood sugar readings, and was already dealing with most of the long-term symptoms of diabetes. A few more years, and he would likely have to deal with amputation of toes and feet and legs, have to deal with vision loss and eventual blindness, perhaps even dialysis and kidney failure. All I needed to do was keep the fat bastard happy, and he would waddle willingly into his own mortality; the eventuality would just take a little more time.

Time.

Why wait?

I opened my eyes and turned my head left to the wall. Even without my glasses in the dim morning light I could see the .45 pistol laying on the nightstand, the pistol my wife had given me the day we got engaged, Valentine's Day. The gift of a gun was such a Southern thing, but it made sense somehow.

How fitting. She doesn't like him, either. Why not have one more bag of Cheetos – there is one in the pantry right now – and then take care of him today? Quick and painless.

Quick. Painless. I could solve so many problems with a single trigger pull. The wife wasn't around, didn't care any more, had abandoned me to stay with family in Memphis under the pretense of caring for a distant family member she hadn't seen in decades. I wasn't happy, hadn't been in years. The marriage was over. No woman really wanted a lard ass son of a bitch like me. I knew we both had settled for what we thought was expedient.

The despair and loneliness were overwhelming. I felt I was sinking to the dark ocean floor as cold numbness enveloped me. I stared at the gun. One simple action. So easy.

I was hurt and angry with myself, angry with my wife's willing participation, angry with the thought that I had handed over control of my life to appetites, squandered the future for instant pleasure. I knew I had done nothing in my life that mattered, nothing more than survive and consume. My obituary played through my mind. "Carl Eugene Moore did little to enhance the human condition and will be mourned by few." Not the legacy I wanted, not what I wanted people to remember me for – merely surviving to eat myself to a premature death. There were so many things I had planned to do in life and, at nearly forty, I had done so few of them. Somewhere along the way from college to working adulthood I had lost the list of dreams and goals I wanted for myself, substituting each one for another 10 pounds of weight and a larger pants size, adding to my sedentary lifestyle in measurable increments. My life had become an exchange of the things and experiences I had wanted for food and entertainment. I was pitiful and I knew it, felt it, and it burned me. The realization that I was nowhere in life and had little of anything to live for hurt. I wanted more. I wanted a life that was more than looking for that next meal, that next fix for a food addict.

I wanted more than what I was and I knew I had finally come to a crossroad and I had to make a decision. I didn't want my obituary to say I was weak and had given up. One thing I knew is that people could change their lives, that goals were achievable if I wanted to work for them. For years I had let everything I wanted fall away unnoticed, wishing for things without wanting to do anything to get them. Sitting in my big recliner was so much easier than jogging. The pain of action was so much greater than inaction and I had taken the inactive road for so long that it was what I knew, comfortable and constant. I had not wanted to expend the energy necessary to pursue my dreams and aspiration so I had let them go and substituted snacks to fill the empty space. That bothered me. I didn't like that I had let food and inactivity rob me of what I wanted out of life. I had to decide if I wanted to continue letting Cheetos have control of my life or if I wanted to take control and begin going after what I wanted. I knew I wasn't weak. I had let my weight take over, fell under the spell of food I loved and handed over my life in exchange. The decision to let that happen may not have been a conscious one, but I was a more than willing participant. I was guilty of gluttony and sloth and apathy. Surviving to eat was not how I wanted to survive any longer.

I felt something stir in me. I wanted more. I wanted to be able to walk a mile. I wanted to be able to jog. I wanted to be able to ride a bike like I did when I was growing up and feel the breeze blowing through what was left of my hair. I didn't want food to have the kind of control over me that it had exercised for too many years. I knew I had issues with food and that I would have to fight to regain ground, but something told me I could. I wanted control. I wanted freedom. I was angry at myself for giving up, for handing over everything I had wanted from life, for letting something outside of me control me. I was angry and embarrassed for thinking about taking an easy way out of something of my own making.

I rolled out of bed, snatched my glasses off the nightstand, and began cursing loudly through the tears, wandering through an empty house looking for nothing, yelling at the furniture, the pictures I hated, the semi gloss Dover White paint that coated every wall, the wife that was always absent in my life.

Realizing the dog was cowering at the back door, I gathered myself, opened the door, and let him out onto the back deck. Morning sun bathed the bleached wood in warm tones that reached across me as I stood in the doorway holding the black metal screen door handle.

Sunday morning and the earth was calm.

Something inside me begged to live. I heard a quiet voice, desperate, yet resolved in some way, reaching out to me in the morning sun through my tears.

You have to fight.

Food was both my dearest friend and most dangerous enemy. I had to eat and often, simply to fuel the biomechanical machine of my body. How was I going to use food instead of it using me?

In my heart, I knew I was not a weak man, but food held me hostage, always there when I needed it. How could I fight something so necessary to life?

I had asked the question – how did I fight – and realized I really had made a decision. Something lifted from my shoulders and I stood a little straighter. I went inside and walked through the house, pacing in and out of each room, for over an hour, trying to get my mind together, trying to work through what I needed to do to get on the road away from where I was.

Food was the issue – what to eat, how much to eat, when to eat. Basic nutrition was simple enough – I knew if I ate more than I could use during the day, the rest would be stored as fat. An increase in physical activity would increase how many calories I needed each day simply to maintain. Easy enough in equation form, but hard to put into practice when the buffet's siren sounded. The journey was not an easy one, but if I was going to live, to beat down the voice that wanted me dead, I had to take the first steps.

I found myself in the kitchen staring into the refrigerator. The shelves were full. I dragged over the trashcan, reached for the first plastic bowl, and opened it: leftover lasagna. Cold noodles and meat made a slapping sound as it hit the bottom of the empty blue trashcan. My favorite leftovers tumbled into the kitchen trash.

When I finished, I had filled both the sink and trashcan; the refrigerator looked almost cavernous. Every high-fat treat I loved – mayonnaise, ranch dressing, whole milk – was trashed. I picked up the heavy, blue Rubbermaid trashcan, hauled it down the back steps, and dumped it in the big, acrid-smelling plastic Herbie Curbie. Then I went back inside to empty the pantry. Three more trips outside and the cupboard was all but bare.

Emptying the fridge and pantry was exhausting, so I flopped in my recliner in the living room and watched Charles Osgood until ten thirty, then got a warm shower. I was hungry when I got out, but refused to go looking for something to eat. When WalMart opened at one-thirty, I went grocery shopping.

I remembered that one of the doctors at my office told his overweight patients always to shop around the perimeter of the grocery store because they could eat pretty much all the foods they found there – raw vegetables, fruits, lean meats, low fat dairy, and one hundred percent whole grains. The other aisles held highly processed foods like snacks and sodas, cookies, canned foods with high sodium content, and other food that contained higher calories and higher fat. The cart I pulled from the rack had a front wheel that whirred and spun constantly as though it were captured in a tiny, isolated tornado. As I pushed it around the store, I tried to remember the doc's advice to select food that would help me get on the right path. Shopping the perimeter of the store was safer, especially for me in trying to restock the house with significantly better choices than I was used to eating. I figured that I could eat all the carrots I wanted without thinking about calories or fat or salt content. I had never heard of anyone getting fat eating pears.

I was scared of food. I started reading the nutrition labels on packaged foods and was overwhelmed. The most disturbing thing about the labels was what the manufacturer considered a serving size and what I considered a serving size. The bag of Cheetos I grabbed on the ride home from work most days and plowed through with deft abandon was designed, according to the people at Frito-Lay, to feed ten people. That meant that I was easily eating at one time the snacks of ten men. Consuming an entire bag, box, can, or platter of anything was what I considered a natural amount of food to eat, single serving size even if it was a two liter soda. Hunger had little to do with it. I always cleaned my plate as a child so cleaning every plate I took from the buffet was ordinary for me and I didn't understand people leaving perfectly good food on their plates. That was wasteful and I grew up in a home where waste was not affordable.

To keep it simple on my first healthy grocery shopping trip, I opted for more fruits and vegetables and items with "fat free" or "low fat" on the label. I thought that was safe. After wearing myself out shuffling around the store behind the grocery cart, I surrendered and went to the checkout.

"Did you find everything ok?" the pale redheaded high school girl working the register asked absently. I mumbled something and started stacking my groceries on the black conveyor belt -- bananas, oranges, apples, cucumbers, tomatoes, 2% cheese slices, low fat mayonnaise, skim milk, fat free turkey breast lunchmeat, fat free hot dogs, diet sodas, fat free cookies, and whole wheat bread. Shopping was not an adventure. I was intimidated, even scared, wanting to make the correct choices. I paid for my groceries and went to the car.

When I got home and put up the groceries, I was ready for a nap. Even that small exertion was enough to wear me out. Realizing that I was so out of shape that even a trip to the grocery store was enough to put me down wasn't easy to swallow, but I caught a nap in the recliner and woke a little more refreshed and in a better, more positive mood.

I struggled out of the recliner then went into the kitchen and ate two bananas and drank a big glass of diet soda. Food was only part of the problem; I knew exercise was the other issue. In high school, I played backyard football and did some haphazard and sporadic weight training, but I was never an athlete and had done virtually nothing resembling exercise in nearly twenty years. My feet, ankles, knees, and hips hurt most of the time, so I avoided even standing when I could. I had never run in my life, though I always wanted to be able to – not a marathon, of course, but a mile, perhaps. In the shape I was in, even a mile was an Everest-like goal, distant and out of reach. I had to start even smaller, measuring progress in steps and minutes instead of miles.

Walking was the best I could hope for at my weight. My doctor had told me over and over that distance walked was not as important as time spent walking. He said to spend thirty minutes every day walking at as brisk a pace as I could manage without getting out of breath. If I couldn't manage thirty minutes at one time, break it up into ten or fifteen minute sessions morning and evening, but get at least thirty minutes daily. I got out of breath simply walking from my office to the bathroom, so I knew that thirty minutes was out of reach. I resolved to do what I could and work from there.

In the middle of a Southern August, there was still light out until late in the evening even after the sun dropped below the horizon. I waited until it was dark before venturing out to my first exercise in two decades. Since I was hot all the time, shorts and large, floppy shirts were in no short supply, and I had headphones and an audio book cassette to listen to while I was walking.

The evening was hot and muggy with the sweet scent of two Russian Tea Olives in bloom coming from up the street. I was already sweating. My shirt stuck to my lower back. I adjusted my headphones, set the volume on the tape player, and stepped slowly down the three concrete steps off the front porch and onto the concrete; then I set out on my walk, already puffing and grunting. I made it all the way to the mailbox at the end of the walkway before getting winded. I turned around and held onto the black plastic box for a couple of minutes, then walked back to the house, hobbled up the steps, went inside, dropped heavily into my recliner, and cried. I was so out of shape that I couldn't even make it past my own mailbox.

Chapter 18

My next slide read "Small Changes."

"If making changes were easy, if we could just start eating right and exercising overnight, we would all be thin and fit and not having this conversation. The reality, of course is that we're all just human and subject to human needs and faults. We do what we do and that usually means we take the easiest path. Exercise every day isn't the easiest path. Making time to walk or to go to the gym is one more thing added to our day. Most of us are already overscheduled and adding an hour of exercise to our daily routine can seem impossible. Realizing this is important and dictates how we approach change, even dramatic lifestyle changes. No one can sustain big changes for long. How many times have you gone on a diet on Monday and realized you stopped that diet by Thursday? We're human. The simple thing is to choose one thing and work on it. I suggest spreading out meals as the first thing to work on. Once spreading out meals becomes a habit, swap out a diet soda a day for a bottle of sugar-free flavored water. Once that's a habit, start looking at portion sizes or calories per serving or lower carbohydrate and higher protein meals, cut back on television time, and get more time in walking. Start with little changes and let them become part of your life before adding more change.

Studies tell us that it takes three weeks to get into a new habit. We can't build a house overnight, we have to take it one brick and one board and one nail at a time. Successful projects, no matter how large, are always broken down into smaller, manageable units. Approach fitness and diabetes management like a project manager. Set attainable, short-term goals – I will go for a thirty minute walk every day this week – and chart your successes."

"Things will change over time. Sure, you will get more fit, but your tastes will change. I used to love a Hardees Thickburger with extra mayo. Now, even the thought of that hunk of cow meat dripping in grease makes me queasy. I can't imagine how I used to take down one of those burgers. I used to drink a six pack of diet soda a day and now I seldom drink soda and can never finish a can of anything. Finding good food and new ways to prepare it is fun, something of a game. Now when I pick up food I read the label and weigh the calorie and carbohydrate and fat costs and decide if I want to eat it. I never go to Chinese buffets any more. Why tempt myself?"

"Does anyone here have regular heartburn?"

Many in the room raised hands.

"I used to have horrible, ongoing heartburn. I would get up and have my morning Alka Seltzer. Then I would have a mid-morning Alka Seltzer. Then I would have yet another in the afternoon. I had heartburn all the time. Let me tell you, since I started eating correctly, I only get heartburn when I overeat and when I eat lots of refined carbohydrates instead of protein. No heartburn. And you know, when I do hit the buffet and overeat and get heartburn, something inside me tells me I deserve it. Wouldn't you like to get off the heartburn meds? Unless you have a medical condition like an ulcer, I would be willing to bet that changing the way you eat will make it better."

Chapter 19

In one of the medical journals in a stack in my hall bathroom, I had read that the majority of heart attacks in the US occur between eight and nine on Monday mornings. There was something about the stress of returning to a job after the weekend off that could trigger a myocardial infarction. There was a 20% increase in the number of heart attacks occurring on Monday morning. Work, it appeared, could kill. Somewhere in my reading, the advice not to begin a diet on a Monday morning appeared, as well, with 31% of Monday diets ending on Tuesday. I had gotten on that Monday morning diet bandwagon enough times to know the truth of that study.

I got dressed, pulling on a pair of black jeans, size 58, and a black XXXL shirt. My work week began with my return to a relatively stressful job, beginning a considerably restrictive diet, and embarking on a new, unfamiliar exercise program, already feeling the soreness of a first, abbreviated foray into walking. Monday coincided with my planned complete change of lifestyle. When I got out of the car in the office parking lot, I was already a mess.

Even though I parked as close to the entrance as possible, I was already sweating by the time I entered the sliding glass front doors, my glasses fogged over from the humidity after nearly an hour of the car's efficient air conditioner on high. August's humid heat was oppressive. The lobby area always reminded me of a water closet, with the horrid choice of little tile squares and the faint, lingering scent of industrial bathroom. A bright silver exhaust fan ran constantly in the middle of the ceiling.

Since Facilities Planning and the building's architect were considerate enough to install an elevator between the first and second floor, I always thought it only equally considerate of me to avail myself of their thoughtfulness. I had ridden the elevator several times a day since we moved into the new building. Knowing that I needed to get more exercise, even in small doses, I decided to swear off the elevator entirely. The fittest coworkers usually used the stairs, parked their cars in the spots most distant from the doors, and brought small-portioned lunches. Stairs meant two flights, one short stretch and one longer stretch above that. I looked at the dull aluminum of the welcoming elevator doors, realized I had made a decision, and then turned to the first set of steps to my right.

I was thirty-six, a professional, and still wore a backpack instead of a laptop bag filled to capacity, slung low on one shoulder. The backpack's shoulder straps were easier for what I carried most days – a heavy laptop, extra cables and power supply, folders and files, cell phone, pda, etc. Laptop shoulder bags never held enough and gave me shoulder and neck pain. The blue and black canvas backpack usually weighed twenty-five or thirty pounds, but the straps over my shoulder distributed the load somewhat more evenly, yet never quite comfortably. The bag was a constant companion that had been with me from Atlanta to Seattle and a myriad of stops between. As I took the first step up, I felt every ounce of laptop and such pulling down on my shoulders. Gravity had never been a friend.

My hands found the round aluminum railing on both sides. I pulled up with each step. The first four steps came slowly. The next four came even more slowly. By the time I reached the first landing, I was out of breath with sixteen more steps ahead of me. I stood there breathing heavily, feeling the backpack press sweat and shirt together against my lower back, and considered walking back down the steps and taking the elevator. The elevator was air conditioned and it would take only seconds to shuttle me from first floor to second. I could always start taking the stairs Tuesday, and who would know?

I would know.

I had made a decision and planned to stay with it. Resolve filled some part of me. I reached for the cool aluminum railing, stepped up, and started hauling myself up the second flight of stairs.

"Mornin', Carl. Elevator broke?" someone asked behind and below me. I stopped three steps up and turned to see one of the secretaries coming up the stairs, a pretty, fit girl with long brown hair and brown eyes trimmed with a shade too much mascara.

"No. Just thought I'd walk up today," I replied, my voice short and breathless. "I could use the exercise," I said forcing a smile.

"Well, just don't overdo it, ok?" she said casually as she passed me. I watched her tight khakis move up the stairs, then followed her slowly, one tiled step at a time. When I finally reached the top of the second flight, I let my backpack slide off my shoulders and onto the floor, then dropped heavily into a brown vinyl chair to rest. At least I was alone in the second floor waiting area, winded and wet, but I had conquered my first obstacle.

Coworkers passed me as they came up the stairs on the way to their offices. Most inquired after my well being. My responses were as cheery as possible as I struggled to regain my breath and some semblance of composure, my lumbar spine damp against distressed vinyl. The clock above the elevator doors noted it was just after eight-thirty. I was late. I was always late.

I had never been an athlete, never been in great shape, even in high school, but at least when I was in my teens, I could walk half a mile without getting so out of breath that I had to sit for ten minutes to recover. I had hiked the Carolina mountains -- Table Rock, Chimney Rock, and Paris Mountain -- when I was the overweight Boy Scout in my troop. In high school, my buddies and I would walk in the evenings the mile or so to the only local convenience store in our one-motorcycle town. Even though I never jogged or ran, I played Sunday afternoon no-blood, no-foul football occasionally. Twenty years of unrestrained eating and lounging in my recliner in front of the television had changed me considerably. I had never realized just how much. Even the thought was depressing. I used to feel young and indestructible even if I was the fat kid waddling in behind everyone else. Somewhere I had lost the young man I continued to think I was. The image of myself carried around in my mind was dramatically different than the chubby reality.

Certainly, I knew I was obese, overweight, big-boned, fat. Sears called me "Husky." That was obvious enough to me from my belt, the wide black leather one I wore that was almost as long as I was tall. Instead of the warning it should have been, the belt and the huge pants and shirts were an amusement, a curiosity, a wellspring of jokes, the huge black slacks run up my high school flagpole when I was in tenth grade. I saw other people as being fat, not me. The bureau mirror I saw myself dressing in each morning distorted reality; that lard ass wasn't me, though I was starting to see more clearly. Somewhere in the pursuit of the trappings of society's ideals of success – the big car, the big TV, the big house, the big meals, I had grown prematurely old and lazy. My leisurely lifestyle was slowly draining me of the ability to enjoy what success I had gained.

I sat recovering for a couple of minutes then hauled myself out of the vinyl chair, reached for my backpack, and walked down the hall to the security door where I waved my magnetic ID badge. The door's electronic solenoid clicked, unlocking the door as I pushed it open and went through. The smell of strong, burned coffee commingled with the acrid smells of a new building that had not quite settled in – paint solvent, industrial carpet adhesive, the mustiness of a sealed environment. As I walked slowly down the hall, I put my hand out to steady myself against the flat beige wall. Ten or twelve steps later, I turned right into my brightly lit outer office.

"Mornin'," I said in greeting to assistant, Bobby. He was sitting in his short-backed blue chair staring into his laptop with a big grin on his face. Computers made the illusion of working so much easier to conjure and maintain.

"Mornin'," he replied without taking his eyes from the electronic source of his amusement. I shook my head and went into my office to the left of his, dropped my backpack into the tan leather chair in front of my desk, went around, and flopped into my own high-backed blue chair. Eight forty-two on a Monday morning and I was already spent and could seriously use a nap.

After I logged in and checked the overnight email, and voice mails, I started a new spreadsheet, naming it

"CM Numbers." From years of working with researchers, I knew that I couldn't measure what I didn't have data for. I needed to start tracking my fasting blood sugar levels, weight, and exercise. If I had a daily accounting of things, I knew I would stick to my goals.

My fasting blood sugar level that morning was 347, a solid 227 points above the top end of the normal range of 80 to 120, bad numbers that I needed to address. My blood sugar was so high that I had headaches most of the day. My glasses prescription would change throughout the day with the increased glucose levels and the resulting higher blood pressure levels it caused. I had never been diagnosed with clinically high blood pressure, but it was always elevated enough to be of long-term concern.

"If I give you anything for it," my doctor had told me several times, "it would knock you on your butt every time you went to stand up. You need to get out and walk," he had said in his biannual lectures to me on my health situation.

Since I had long since outgrown the home bathroom scale that went all the way up to 280 pounds, I had no idea what I weighed. However, the practice had two hyper-accurate in-floor scales in the patient care areas. I didn't remember seeing a weight limit on them, but I knew we had some Toyota-sized patients who we had weighed on them. Once the morning patient care had settled, I could go down and weigh myself for the first time in perhaps ten years.

Walking, I knew, would be measured in steps and time, not miles. Several of the office staff, some who needed to drop 20 or 30 pounds, had made a short-lived effort to wear belt-clipped pedometers to record daily and weekly walking progress both in steps and miles. Like most half-hearted, unreinforced initiatives, the program died sometime around the second week and we had a big box of pedometers left over from the initiative. I wandered around to the supply closet, and liberated one for my own use. I planned to use it to account for my daily walking. When I got back to my office I tossed it on the desk.

Bobby came into my office around nine. We usually met each morning after we both had caught up to discuss where tasks were and what we needed to work on that day and the rest of the week.

"So, what's up?" he asked as he pushed my backpack aside and dropped into the tan leather chair in front of my desk.

"Not a hell of a lot," I said not looking away from my monitor.

Bobby and I had been friends for years. A mutual friend of ours called one Saturday afternoon in November of 1993, just after I had lost my job. He was working on Bobby's computer and having problems with it. Whatever the issue was, I couldn't diagnose it over the phone, so I told him to pack up the hardware and send Bobby to my house, and I would see what I could do.

I was in the yard when a little two-tone Chevy S-10 pickup turned into the driveway next to my Town Car. The passenger front tire rubbed against the inside of the truck's fender, making a nasty, hollow, rubber-on-metal growl. The truck wasn't two-tone in the sense of the top half was one color and the bottom a different, complimentary color. The cab was white and the long bed was cream, the paint flat and oxidized where it wasn't rusted or where chunks of sheet metal was missing. The bed was filled with all manner of tools, parts, and the unidentifiable.

I saw Bobby's dirty black ball cap over the top of the truck before I saw him – soiled dark green service uniform with his name over the left breast pocket, black sneakers with the shoelaces trailing, hands black with ground-in grease and dirt up past both elbows. Shoulder-length black hair sprouted barely restrained from under his dirty cap, his face framed with lots of black beard, mustache, and sideburns. There was an easy smile in there somewhere, a young, hillbilly Santa who worked as a mechanic in the off season. I didn't know what to think.

I was able to fix Bobby's computer problem, making a permanent friend in the process. He had just quit his job and I was out of work at the time, too, so we started spending lots of time together. He introduced me to hobby shops and the finer junkyards in the area. We were inseparable, though we had little in common. We made an unusual pair riding around in my shiny Lincoln all over South Carolina, North Carolina, and Georgia. When it snowed in December, he taught me to do doughnuts in a Service Merchandise parking lot in the big, rear wheel drive car.

Bobby was lean and strong from years of physical labor with his hands. He was skilled in all manner of skilled labor from carpentry to mechanical work and seemed to know almost everything about how the physical world functioned in the same way I knew technology. We both ate fast food two or three times a day, snacks in between, getting in a buffet regularly, though it took outright coercion to get him into a Chinese restaurant the first few times. His wife, Michelle, was surprised I had gotten him to even try Chinese food, but he came to enjoy it. Years of turning wrenches and pounding hammers gave him a metabolism that could burn off whatever he ate, so he never gained weight while working those jobs. I continued to eat the way I had with even less daily exertion. Soon my black jeans were getting tighter. Bobby never openly judged me.

Eventually I got Bobby out of the uniforms, got him to quit wearing the ball cap everywhere, and cut the shoulder-length hair to a reasonable level. He picked up technology quickly and soon I found him a job with a vendor who owed me a litany of favors. When my network assistant left for a better job with the local school district, we hired Bobby.

"Get a pedometer?" he asked reaching for the package. Then he carved around the pedometer with a green, plastic-handled #10 scalpel. Our nurse manager kept him supplied in all manner of disposable medical equipment he re-tasked for more mundane purposes such as opening boxes. When he had extricated the black plastic pager-like device, he tossed the package into the trash, and then set the pedometer back on my desk.

"You gonna start using that?" he asked.

"Plan to. I went for a short walk last night," I said, leaving out the particulars of how short a walk it really was.

"That's great," he said. "Me and Michelle need to start getting out and walkin' up the dirt road every day. But our knees just hurt so much and that gravel just makes it worse. And it gets dark earlier now and who knows what's in those woods and all. Michelle can get a cheap family membership at the Y and I think maybe we're going to start doin' that maybe start of the year. We could go up there a couple of times a week and walk around in the pool and stuff."

I knew he meant it, but also knew exercise wasn't a priority in that house.

When I first met Bobby, he weighed about 185. A few years of sitting in the office, and he had worked his way up to 255. He may have disliked exercise even more than I did. His diet was certainly no better.

"I'm gonna start walking every day," I said.

"That's great. Really. You need to start getting out and walking. It's good for you. You know, if we still lived in town, we could come up in the evening and walk with you. That would be nice. But when we get home and get settled, I don't want to drive back into town. You know. I mean by the time we get in and get settled and eat dinner, it's time for our shows and then it's time for bed. Really just no time to do much after work."

Bobby was a big boy, too, and I knew he was not spending much time walking and wouldn't if he lived in town. I was resolute.

"Yeh, well, I'm going to start making time. I have to." There was a finality in the statement; I was trying to convince the both of us that walking was going to become part of my life.

We talked about the work day and what we needed to focus on for the week. Then he left to get started on his list for the day. I knew patient care would be well underway and the scales would be free. I left my office, opened the door to the back stairwell, and started down the steps. My ankles and knees, especially my right knee, hurt most of the time, so I took the stairs slowly, deliberately, paying attention to the joint pain. Going down the stairs was in many ways tougher than going up them. My full weight landed on each foot, the jolt traveling up my ankles, into my knees, into my hips, and ultimately into my lower back. My feet were numb from diabetic neuropathy, almost like the mountain climber with frozen feet, so I had to get both visual and pressure indications to make sure I landed squarely on each step. Descending stairs had its own issues, but was far easier than walking up them. I was careful, held tightly to the railing, and wished for an escalator.

I made it down both flights, went through the door at the bottom of the stairs, and turned left into the patient care area. I walked past several nurses at the long nursing counter, exchanged morning pleasantries, then turned right into the empty vitals room. Mounted in the floor close to one wall was a stainless steel platform four feet by four feet, large enough to accommodate motorized wheelchairs. An aluminum panel with red numbers in the display was set in the wall. I stepped on the platform and watched the numbers spin up like I had spun a game show wheel and was waiting to see what my prize was. I had not weighed in years, so I had no idea what to expect, but big numbers were not welcome. Five seconds passed before the bright red numbers read 387. I was only 13 pounds from weighing 400, not much more than a good day's eating.

If I had not felt depressed from the tough trip up the stairs that morning, the knowledge that I weighed almost a quarter of a ton instantly dissolved any positive things the morning may have brought. Almost 400lbs. I was well into the journey to becoming the guy who weighed 1000lbs, the guy I never thought I could be, never wanted to be.

A nurse went to the door near me and called out a name to patients in the waiting room. I would need to leave the vitals room. I got off the scale and walked past her to the elevator and pushed the white square button. The doors opened immediately and I stepped inside to wait for them to close once more. Before they did, I saw one of our young male residents start up the stairs two steps at a time. The dull silver elevator doors closed.

I wanted to be him.

Chapter 20

When I was trying out for Junior Varsity football in eighth grade, I made an attempt at lifting weights with the other guys in my class, but it was something I did occasionally, more a social activity than exercise to lose weight and build muscle. As an adult, I knew nothing about resistance training; once again, I consulted the library, this time online. I did a few internet searches on fitness and weight loss and found a web site with strength training exercises with pictures and descriptions of exercises and muscle groups they targete, information I could work with. Weighing as much as I did limited what I could do, and I knew I wasn't going to walk into a gym and start bench pressing a Mazda Miata. I had to start slow and small if for no other reason than to keep from injuring myself. I couldn't afford a trainer, so it would be up to me to get started and develop a routine over time. I made a short list of things I thought I could do and tucked the printed pages of exercises into my backpack.

On the way home, I didn't stop for snacks. Stopping at convenience stores was off my list as were fast food restaurants. I knew I couldn't handle a buffet so I stayed away from them as well. As with cleaning out the refrigerator and pantry at home, I knew I had to keep from bringing mass quantities of food into my life that prevented me from reaching my goals. Fast food and cheesy, salty snacks provided no health value for an addict trying to crawl out of a fat-wrapped hell and I meant to avoid them whenever possible.

That evening I had what I considered a sensible, low fat meal. In quantity. Part of my problem was that I had stretched out my stomach so that it simply took more food to make me feel full. I couldn't sit down to a meal and eat a normal serving of food. Even in diet mode, I was eating three or four times what I should, but at least I wasn't covering everything in Duke's mayonnaise or sharp cheddar. That alone counted for a significant calorie and fat gram reduction even if I was still packing in more than I should. I didn't know what the measurement was, but if I was eating 500 or 1000 calories fewer a day, I considered it significant progress. I had to start somewhere in manageable steps.

After dinner, I changed into a pair of grey sweat pants and a huge powder pink and blue shirt I'd had for years and sat on the couch watching television and looking at the exercise sheets I had printed at the office. Exercise was so foreign to me. I selected two body weight exercises I thought I could do at home and do regularly. "Body weight" meant I didn't need weights or a machine or anything to get started and I didn't have to go somewhere public. The latter was a major consideration. Just like walking, I didn't want to be seen, so I walked after dark.

Pushups were first on my list. I had done pushups in junior high PE class, but I hadn't pushed up off anything since eighth or ninth grade. Certainly, I would never be able to do a full guy pushup, a Marines pushup, but I thought I would be able to start out doing girl pushups, knees bent with my shins on the floor. I knew I was starting my climb at he very bottom of the fitness ladder and I my first goal was that first rung – just one pushup of any kind to start.

Actually getting down and on the carpet was tough enough. My creaking, cracking knees were less than cooperative and my hips hurt from years of walking around with that much weight, but I got down in the floor in front of the couch and assumed proper pushup position, my chubby arms wide and palms flat to the floor. My black lab slid off the couch and wandered over to see what I was doing, his big, wet nose sniffing mine.

"It's ok, Son, Daddy's exercising."

He must have understood because he stretched into a long forward bow, yawned with his long red tongue curling up, then flopped down on the blue carpet in front of me to watch through heavy eyelids.

I pushed against the floor and the floor pulled back. Hard. I made it up and held the moment, then dropped quickly back to the carpet. I pushed again, made it to the top, then dropped quickly back to earth. A third pushup was the end of the exercise. I had made it through three complete girl pushups. Lying on the carpet recovering, I looked into my Lab's brown eyes until he closed them and started snoring.

I was more successful with squats. When I got out of the floor, I went to stand behind one of the chairs. Holding onto the back of the couch, I slowly bent my knees into a squat then pushed up until I was standing straight. I was able to squat holding onto the back of the couch ten times before I was winded and sweaty. Everything from my hips down complained, but I made it into an almost sitting position before moving back to the top of the squat. Naturally, my legs were already weightlifting all day from when I got out of bed until I went back to bed, so I had huge calf muscles from carrying around the weight, just very little stamina. My cardiovascular system was wearing out long before my leg muscles. I was walking every night, too, so my leg muscles were in much better shape for hauling the rest of me around.

I slept well that night, better than in recent memory, but I felt something new. I was sore. At first, it was just enough around the edges to notice, but by lunchtime I was starting to hurt. By the time I left work, I could feel the previous night's activity in my shoulders, chest, and back of my legs. After I ate a sensible supper, I came close to talking myself out of a walk, but I kept to it. By the time I had reached the end of the street, I my lower body wasn't hurting at all, so I continued my walk. When I got home, I got back in the floor and did three pushups, then eight squats at the back of the couch. Lying in bed that night, I didn't notice any soreness as all as I drifted right off to a restful sleep that hadn't visited me in years.

*

Every night I tried to get a walk in. I knew daily aerobic exercise was the best thing for managing my blood sugar and I could tell the following morning when I checked my blood sugar if I hadn't walked. After the first night's walk all the way to the mailbox, I had gone back out the second night and made it to my mailbox and halfway to the neighbor's mailbox. The next night I made it all the way to the neighbor's mailbox. Within a week, I was walking all the way up the small hill next to my house and down the hill to Main Street, a milestone for me having not walked much in perhaps twenty years. After two weeks, I was able to make it all the way around my block and within the month I could make the whole two block area around my house, hill and all, without feeling like a fellow climber had stolen my last oxygen bottle before summiting Everest.

Resistance training showed comparable progress as I made an effort to do pushups and squats every night.

Floor pushups were simply too tough for my weight, so I stood at an angle against a wall in the living room and began doing pushups, or push outs, against the wall. The first time I tried the wall method, I was able to get six. In a couple of weeks, I could do an even dozen. When I reached twenty, I placed my feet farther out, making a steeper and harder incline against the wall. When I got to the point I could do twenty at that angle, I increased the angle and kept at it until I could get in the floor and do a dozen girl pushups without passing out. Similarly, I was able to work my way up to more than one set of twenty or twenty five squats holding onto the back of the couch to stabilize myself and my joints complained less.

My workouts began to get easier and I actually began looking forward to trying something new or trying to get one or two more squats or pushups more than I had done the previous session. As out of shape as I was, I began to see results quickly. I could go a little longer, go a little further, do a little more without getting worn out nearly as quickly. I was seeing progress and progress felt good.

*

I pulled on my faded black jeans for work one Monday morning and they seemed to be more room in them than I was used to. I threaded my long, black leather belt into the loops, cinched it up, and noticed the latch fell naturally into the second hole instead of the stretched-out first one. While I couldn't see a difference in the mirror, my jeans fit better. I pulled on a shirt and it seemed to fit less snug as well. When I got to the office, I went down and stepped on the scales. The numbers showed I had lost five pounds, but I was sure I was down a pants size. I wasn't going to argue, I had lost weight and could tell it.

Over the next two months, my pants and belt continued to slowly grow. Coworkers noticed the change and complimented me. While the attention was embarrassing, I did take pleasure in it. I kept up my nightly walking. When I took the stairs at work, I no longer felt like I was tempting a myocardial event, and could make both flights without stopping, though I was still a bit winded when I reached the second floor.

What I found was that I couldn't just go out walking at night for pleasure or exercise, I had to have a reason to go for a walk. The books on tape I bought off eBay and borrowed from the local library helped pass the time, but walking wasn't a pleasurable experience, walking was exercise and didn't entertain the way sitting on the couch flipping through seventy channels of cable on a sixty inch television did. Fortunately, I had several retail establishments within a mile of my house, located off the Main Street sidewalk at the end of my street, and soon were within my walking ability. I began looking at my weekly grocery list, walking to Walmart, buying two or three items on the list, then walking home with them. I began walking to Blockbuster to rent and return movies and CVS to refill my long list of monthly medications. Those errands gave me purpose and reason to be out walking every night and made a huge difference in my motivation. Being out for an hour every night also gave me time to think, to let my mind wander in a way it didn't at work or in front of the television. I bought my first iPod, loaded it with music from my large CD collection, and started listening to music I hadn't heard in years, music from high school and college, and albums long misplaced. In time, I began to find myself looking forward to getting home and lacing up the walking shoes and getting out of the house. I began feeling the need for that time alone with myself and missed it when the rain was too much or I simply got home too late in the evening. Walking became part of my routine.

I weighed almost every day at the office. After two months of walking and strength training at home, I had lost 35 pounds and dropped two pants sizes. My morning blood sugars showed similar results as the numbers began to come down almost daily. My usual reading of 350 quickly dropped to 300, then to 275. I was beating the disease.

Chapter 21

"This is big," I said to the audience. "You have to love yourself. I found love in food for most of my life and food never returned that love. If you love someone, you treat them well, you want to see them happy and content, and sometimes you hold back or whip their behind out of love. Fitness and your health are no different. If you don't love you, then you'll cram Cheetos and cheese fries down all day with disregard for your long term happiness."

"Frankly, after years of that kind of self-abuse, I really hated myself, so I crammed even more food down to try to make that hurt go away. That didn't help. I felt worse. But once I started caring about me, looking after me, taking myself out for a walk and weightlifting, I started to really feel better, feel good about myself. That changes things. My personality changed. I used to be introverted. You wouldn't know that now. I love to be seen now and I can talk all day about this to thirty or thirty thousand."

"There is, of course, the potential or the problem that diet and exercise isn't enough and this brings up other personality issues. Often fat people have packed on weight to get away from something. I don't want to get too close to home for anyone here, but there are psychological issues that may need to be addressed – depression, trauma, abuse, stress. Certainly being fit and healthy will help you deal with these issues better, but you may still need to see someone to talk through some of this. These things are outside my area of expertise. I can tell you I booked couch time with one of the psychs I work with and some of that helped me. But I tell you, being in better shape worked wonders that talking with someone about my childhood didn't."

I changed the slide to show the magazine covers of *Women's Health* and *Men's Health* magazines with extremely fit cover models on them. There was a collective chuckle in the room. I'd titled the slide "Reasonable Expectations."

"Folks," I begin with a laugh of my own, "I'm sorry, but you just aren't going to look like that," I say pointing at the screen. "For that matter, they don't look like that in real life. That's a social ideal, retouched photographs. These people are what our society thinks is the epitome of good looks. That ideal represents less than one percent of the earth's population, but accounts for something like ninety-eight percent of television and movies. There just aren't a lot of fat, ugly people on television. If there are, the character is either a bumbling clown or a villain. You have to set goals for yourself, your body image, but you also have to be realistic. The outdated body weight charts say I should weigh in about 185 and no more. Personally, I think I would look terrible at 185. One of my coworkers started exercising and dieting here recently and lost a lot of weight. Now he's so gaunt people started asking if he was sick. I want a happy medium. My goal is around 220 with my body type. And if I can maintain a low A1c and low blood pressure and low cholesterol at 220, that's where I'll do my best to maintain. Besides, I don't think the editors at *Men's Health* are going to be calling me for a cover shoot."

Chapter 22

My local Walmart sold jeans up to a size 50, as if fat people didn't shop there. I never understood that because a quick review of the customers in the store at any time of day would indicate otherwise. I had lost enough weight that I had to buy new jeans, the old ones were so baggy and hard to keep up that I looked like I was playing dress up in them. I walked to Walmart one evening and went directly to the jeans section. I reached down to the bottom shelf and selected the largest pair of black Wranglers I could find, size 50, "Relaxed Fit," and took them to the dressing room. I slid out of my black sweat shorts and pulled on the jeans. They buttoned. Even though they were at least eight inches too long, they fit. I rolled the extra material up on each leg and stood there looking at myself in the full-length mirror. The jeans fit. I had walked to the retail rack in a store that didn't carry "fat clothes," got a pair of name brand jeans off the shelf, put them on, and they actually fit!

I walked home with two pair.

*

I bought a pair of 5 pound dumbbells and started branching out into more weightlifting exercises at home. When 5 pounds wasn't enough, I bought a set of 10 pound weights and started working with them. After a few weeks, I was working with 10 pounds easily enough and knew it was time to start considering a gym.

"You know that faculty and staff can use the university gym for free," a coworker commented one day. No, I didn't know, but that was welcome news if it was true. I really couldn't afford a gym membership and I hadn't even been in one since high school. When I looked up the school's gym web page, I learned that I could indeed use all of the gym's facilities free of charge by showing my university ID. The facility was across town, but not seriously out of the way for me. I could leave the office and be there in about ten minutes if traffic wasn't against me, so I decided to try out the facilities.

Monday morning I left the house in a new pair of jeans my mother had cut off and hemmed over the weekend and a blue nylon bag for my shorts, t-shirt, and walking shoes. That was a first; I had never taken my walking clothes anywhere.

There was a certain level of excitement and fear that stayed with me all day. Not only was going to a gym a new experience, this was a university gym where young athletes worked out. Fit college students would surround me. Going into a gym with a bunch of reasonably fit people my age would have been tough enough, but I planned to exercise in public with people nearly half my age and most of them in the best shape of their lives – football players, soccer players, cheerleaders, and average students without anything close to a weight problem, young, beautiful people for the most part, the popular kids.

At 4:30, I closed my door and changed in the privacy of my own office into my "workout clothes," black shorts, a black muscle shirt, and white sneakers. Even being in shorts and a sleeveless shirt as I walked through the hall at the office was new and made me slightly nervous. Something about the bare arms felt good; I felt like I was really part of the population who left work at the end of the day to exercise.

I walked to the car and drove across town. Though I had never actually been in the PE Center gym, I knew where it was on campus. Some years earlier, I worked just up the hill from the PE Center and watched students playing on the surrounding fields during breaks from the break room balcony overlooking them. Often I wanted to be one of them, a lean, strong athlete running from one end of the field to the other simply for the joy of being outside playing in the summer sun with friends. I had never run in my life and had no expectation of ever being able to. I genuinely wanted to run. I wanted to kayak. I wanted to be normal, not a guy wearing a lard overcoat all the time.

Classes were in session, so the parking lot in front of the PE Center and the parking spaces on the road were mostly taken. I almost gave up and drove away, but found an open spot near the gym and parallel parked. I sat in the car with the air conditioner cranked up and the radio on. Fit college students were walking the sidewalks and they were all young and lean and nothing like me. I watched several go into the gym. I began to get nervous and self-conscious. Though I hadn't checked a mirror, I could imagine what I looked like stretching out my shirt and shorts, and how I looked waddling across the street. I could imagine the thoughts of others around me as I tried to lift weights.

Damn, who let the lardass in here?

Doesn't he know what he looks like?

I thought the gym was just for students. Who let the old, fat guy in?

The voices of their thoughts were clear and distinct in my head, and worse comments floated through. I sat paralyzed in the car as the cold air blew against me. That little voice in my head came forward after a while telling me that there was a beginning for everything, that first step on the journey, and getting past my fear and embarrassment was one such first step that I had to make. I had to get through that initial fear and just get into those double doors. That was my small victory for the day. I made the decision to follow through and go inside.

The sun was shining directly into the car's front window so I unfolded the silver sunshade and stuck it in the window against the heat. Then I turned off the car, opened the door, and stepped out in to the muggy afternoon. I could smell the hot asphalt under my feet and feel the sun on my bare arms and face. After I looked both ways up and down the street, I walked across to the opposite sidewalk and started toward the glass double doors.

As I walked past the drink machines and half-filled bike rack, a girl began to exit the gym. I reached out and grabbed the big brass handle and held one of the doors open for her. She was beautiful, looked like she had just wrapped a photo shoot with a surfing magazine. The girl was thin and fit with long, black hair still wet from the pool or a shower, sunglasses, and a blue print beach towel wrapped around her waist. I held the door for her and smiled and she looked through me as if I was little more than a transparent doorman, an expected, unnoticed fixture. She breezed past me and I stood holding the door much longer than necessary before going in.

I was used to women ignoring me, acting like I wasn't even in the room. That didn't make it any easier when it happened, especially when the girl was as beautiful as miss surfer girl, but there was little I could do about it. The couple of times I had the nerve or frustration to say something, they usually ignored me even more, so I let it go. Fat people are amazingly invisible to the beautiful people.

I walked in and handed my ID card to the student working the desk. He didn't look up from his textbook as he swiped my card and handed it back.

"Where is the weight room?" I asked.

He pointed down the hall, "second floor. Take the stairs to the left up two flights."

I wandered off in the direction he had pointed. The concrete block walls were painted in an off-white cream color and covered with printed sheets advertising for exercise buddies, kayaking clubs, yoga classes, and all manner of social collegiate activity, events I had missed out on during my college days.

The stairs were steep and intimidating and there wasn't an elevator. I had to pull along the round, steel rails to steady myself to get up both flights. Two tall basketball players breezed past me on their way to the court above. I got to the second floor and looked into one door to see the basketball court, the other door showed a carpeted floor inside. I entered to find a huge weight room, a converted basketball court, the scoreboards still affixed to the walls and hoop backboards pulled back and up out of the way. The walls were all mirrored and there were racks of free weights down both sides. New, white machines were in rows with middle areas for stretching and floor mats. Young people were everywhere with earbuds hanging from their ears. I took their cue and plugged in my own earbuds and turned on my iPod and tried to remain invisible.

In health clubs, there is usually someone who will take the new member on a tour, answer questions, and often offer an attended first workout to get the new member oriented to what the gym has to offer. The university gym was staffed by two work-study students who sat at a desk reading textbooks. I was on my own.

The free weights I understood, but most of the machines were a mystery. I watched people using some of them to get an idea of how they worked. Fortunately, most of the machines had a graphic on them with the machine's name and a picture of a man with what muscle groups were targeted colored in red or orange, and some suggestion of the range of motion the machine was supposed to move in. As I looked at the graphics on each machine, I realized they were separated more or less into the major muscle groups – arms, shoulders, back, legs, and so on throughout the huge room. I had read that people who "hit the gym" four or five days a week work on different muscle groups each day, I decided I would try to do the same. On Monday, I would work on upper body, Tuesday I would work on lower body, Wednesday I would rest and get on the treadmill or elliptical, Thursday I would work on upper body again, then Friday would be a lower body day. I wanted to start building lean body mass – muscles – as quickly as possible.

The first weight machine I approached, the one closest to the door, was a chest press. I went around to each side and struggled to hang a large, black 45 pound round steel plate on each side of the machine. Most everyone seemed to be using the big black plates, so I went with them not knowing what an appropriate weight was for me for any of the machines. I sat down, adjusted the seat, and assumed what I considered to be the proper position. My hands wrapped naturally around the foam-covered handles and pushed hard, but the weight pushed back much harder. The weight I selected was clearly too much for me. I got up and took off the big plates and hung two 25 pound plates on the machine and sat back down. When I pushed against the handles a second time, the weight relented, and I was able to get ten reps before tiring. I was sweating and a little winded, but the sensation wasn't unpleasant. I rested a couple of minutes and went for another set of ten. The weight was a little lighter and I wasn't as winded when I completed the set.

Some of the other young people around me looked at me now and then, but none stared that I noticed. I assumed they were watching me when I wasn't looking. While I was extremely self-conscious, the exertion, the concentration, kept me occupied. There simply wasn't any way to press with all my strength against steel weights and pay attention to what others were doing in the room. What I had read of the proper form when lifting weights said I needed to control my breathing, breathe deeply and out as I pushed the weight, then breathe deeply and in as I lowered the weight. With trying to coordinate pressing and breathing and making a real effort not to hyperventilate, I was pretty well occupied.

I rested for another couple of minutes before moving on to the next machine, a similar station with the handles at a different angle to work the chest muscles in a slightly different angle. I chose another two 25 pound plates and was able to get through two more sets. I continued through three more upper body machines before tiring to the point I felt I couldn't keep at it. I wiped the sweat off my head and neck and started for the stairs back down to the first floor.

The stairs seemed even steeper looking down and I felt a little lightheaded. The height and deep breathing got to me. I grabbed the railing and slowly stepped down both flights to the floor below. I could already feel my shoulders tightening, knew I was going to hurt the next day. I hadn't yet read about stretching after weightlifting.

The walk back to the car felt shorter than the walk in. I felt bigger, stronger, even though I could tell my real strength was nearly spent. By walking into a public gym and working out with college athletes in great physical shape, I had crossed a threshold. When I got home, I plugged in my earbuds, turned on my iPod, and went for a walk in the sun.

That night I slept well, "the sleep of the just." After work the next day, I was back in the gym working on lower body exercises. I took note of the graphics on the various leg machines and put weight on each until it became challenging – squats, leg extensions, calf extensions, leg press – enough to wear me out quickly. On the leg press, I could easily get ten reps out with five 45 pound plates on each side, a total of 450 pounds. As my legs had been pressing serious weight every day of my life, I had finally found something I could do that at least looked impressive. When I moved to the inclined squat rack and started hanging 45 pound steel plates, several of the big guys around me took notice.

By the time I felt I had worked out enough and went to leave, I had to hold onto the metal rails with both hands to hobble down the steep stairs, but I kept giggling through the weakness in my leg muscles and the giddy, lightheaded feeling. Coming down the stairs, I thought I knew something of what was called "runner's high" where endorphins are released to deal with physical pain and strain from endurance exercises. Since my fitness level was still so incredibly low, especially compared to any of the college athletes I was working out with, hitting the threshold of "endurance exercise" wasn't all that tough for me. I knew the soreness wasn't going to be fun the next couple of days. I was right.

Working out by myself with no direction meant I had to learn as I went. The next day I simply hurt too much all over to consider going to the gym, but Wednesday was my chosen day off during the week, so when I got home that afternoon, I walked up to Blockbuster to rent a movie. The round trip was just over two miles and I knew stretching my legs would help with the soreness. The lactic acid buildup in my muscles that caused soreness would go away much more quickly if I stayed in motion, kept the hurting muscles working a little to push the lactic acid out of the muscle. A walk was exactly what I needed.

"I can tell you're losing weight," the clerk at Blockbuster commented. Since I was in the store so often and she knew I was out walking, she had seen my progress over time.

"Yeh, I'm at about 35 pounds so far. Coupla pants sizes. Just started getting serious about weightlifting at the gym."

"Really? That's great. I've been thinking about joining the gym downtown on Main Street. You know the one in the old Belks building."

I knew the one, walked past it every time I walked all the way downtown and to Nance Street and back. I also knew she was talking without planning any doing. I talked a lot, too, but I was following through on the doing aspect of things, actually getting out every day for a walk and going to the gym.

When I got home from my walk, my back and underwear were wet as usual. I went straight to the kitchen and got a container of 2% Walmart cottage cheese out and started eating it with a spoon while drinking diet lemonade. I used to absolutely hate cottage cheese of any percentage, but since I had started getting serious about exercise, I couldn't get enough of the 2% variety. Fortunately, from my reading, I knew that low fat cottage cheese was something of a perfect food, something that bodybuilders and people who lost large amounts of weight and kept it off ate in copious quantities. I was fortunate in that I truly liked it. Sometimes I would fill a bowl with cottage cheese and golden raisins and cinnamon. Sometimes I would mix it with warm salsa. Even plain was just fine with me. I tried to eat a few large spoons just before bed each night to keep something low fat and high protein in my stomach overnight.

Over time, I found my tastes in food changing. I used to love Duke's mayonnaise to the point that I could sit down with a jar of Duke's, a loaf of white bread, and a pack of cheese slices, and just eat mayo and cheese sandwiches. I had done similar things growing up, often adding thick-sliced bologna to the sandwich menu. I could easily eat through a quart jar of Duke's in a week – the creamy oil, egg, salt mixture so tangy-delightful on my tongue. Sometimes I would dip sharp cheddar cheese slices directly in the mayo or spread on French's yellow mustard and eat most of a block of cheese that way standing in the kitchen. I loved cheese, loved high fat and creamy food. For me, salads were little more than Ranch Dressing Delivery Systems – the wetter, the better.

Something happened, though, as I started exercising and pushing my body to do things daily that went beyond sitting on the couch watching television every evening. I began eating less mayonnaise, less Ranch dressing, and less cheese. I began wanting more cottage cheese, more diet drinks and less sugar-filled snacks. My love affair with Cheetos waned somewhat, though I never stopped loving the crunchy orange goodness. What I found, though, was that I started putting what I thought about eating in a mental balance. I weighed the long term cost of eating a cheese and mayo sandwich on white bread with how it would make me feel later in the day, with how it would turn into long term fat around my belly or thighs. When I started seeing these foods in context, as a cost factor, as a sort of financial balance sheet, I started asking myself if I really wanted Cheetos or half a block of cheese and mayo as a late night snack. When I started putting these questions to myself, the answer began coming up "no" more often than not. I wasn't hungry or wasting away. I was getting plenty of food and feeling full and enjoying playing the new game, the game of "do I really want this" or not. When I started making more conscious decisions, I started eating less of the things that packed on the weight.

Cheese and mayonnaise and Cheetos still called to me, but I kept them out of the house. If I didn't buy them, I couldn't just walk into the kitchen and eat them. That was simple for me and I needed things simple, needed a simple plan to follow that became part of my life.

Chapter 23

My last slide was titled "Your Health Care is YOUR Problem."

"Ok, folks, here is the 'takeaway' as they say in some of my business meetings. All of what I have said to you today is important, but this is what I want you to leave with today. Like the slide says, your health care is your concern and yours alone. You may have someone who loves you and looks after you, but you are the one responsible for your health, your fitness, your well being. You are the one who has to decide if you want to eat that double cheeseburger and extra large fries for lunch or the grilled chicken salad with low fat dressing on the side route. You are the one who has to motivate yourself to get out for a thirty-minute walk after dinner every evening. You have to manage your health. First, you need to know all of your numbers and get them updated regularly. If you don't know your number, you can't access your health and develop a plan to address what needs improvement.

As a Diabetic, you should have at least one A1c a year. I try to get an A1c three times a year so I have more recent information to work from. You need your blood pressure and cholesterol checked regularly, too. And you should know every medication you are on and what the dosage is for each one. Keep a notebook and take that notebook with you to every doctor's visit along with your list of questions. You have to understand that it is not your doctor's job to keep up with your life. Just like with your mechanic, you take your body in for maintenance or to be fixed when it's broke.

Does your doctor come to your house every morning after breakfast to make sure you take the correct dose of your medication? No. My doctor has been my primary care doc for almost seventeen years. Since he was my boss for many of those years, he knows so much more about me than he does most of his patients. I was having lunch with him one day and asked him about something and he turned to me and said, 'Now, what are you on again?'

Why should he remember? He may see sixteen patients in a morning or afternoon in patient care. How can he possibly keep up with each individual's medication list? No, YOU are the one who is responsible for you. Take that job seriously. Take care of you."

I clicked for the next slide, but the screen went black.

*

"Ok, folks, I've talked on and on. Please feel free to hit me with questions."

Hands reached for air before I finished the sentence.

"Yes," I said pointing.

"Which diet is the best one?" came from the audience.

"That's easy. They ALL work. And NONE of them work. Sure, I'm being flip, but I want to make a point. We all want to know which diet works best and the secret is that they all can work for the most part. There is a journey we each have to take to find out which diet is best for us. What works for you may not work as well for me. Maybe my body won't react to it or maybe it just doesn't fit my lifestyle. I don't know about you, but I don't want to stand in the kitchen every night fixing hummus and potato chip casseroles or something else weird. Frankly, I don't have that kind of time. The important thing is to try a diet for a while, give it a month so you have a chance to settle into it, and chart your results before deciding if it works for you. When you do find a diet or program that fits you, STICK WITH IT! We are human. We have a tendency to 'fall off the wagon' as they say. Consistency will give you long-term results. Stick with your program."

"Ok, I know you want some specifics," I continued, "and I'll try to oblige without becoming a product spokesman. If I had to choose one diet for diabetics, The *South Beach Diet* looks really good. *South Beach* is a low carbohydrate approach that is tested and manageable over time."

I could see Amy nodding her approval.

"I know plenty of people have lost weight on Atkins, but I've been diabetic too long to give my kidneys any more stress than they need and the Atkins program or any all-protein diet has got to be tough on your kidneys with the forced ketosis the diet tries to get your body into. I am a big fan of the *Body for Life* program, especially for those starting out who have never been into strength training and cardio programs. The book contains inspirational stories, meal plans, weightlifting plans, examples of exercises, and you can find the book cheap on eBay and Amazon. I like it for inspiration and basic planning. There's also the *ABS Diet* from the folks who publish *Men's Health, Women's Health, Best Life*. If you are already in decent shape or used to be in good shape and workout, the *ABS Diet* may be great, but it's not for beginners."

Someone in the audience asked, "any other advice on which foods to eat? Especially packaged foods?"

"Sure. We all know fruits and vegetables. But who wants to eat carrots all day? During World War II, British pilots were fed carrots so often that their skin had a tendency to take on an orange tint from all the beta-carotene. We have to plan eating around our industrialized lives. So, I suggest snacks such as mixed nuts. I have to have some salt in mine, so I buy a can of unsalted and a can of lightly salted and mix them. I also stash cheap peanut butter in my office. And I make up pint Mason jars of instant oatmeal with Splenda and dried fruit and nuts and eat it right out of the jar after workouts on the way home. Great snack."

I took a few similar questions before Amy stood and came to the front of the room.

"One more question," she said.

"Do you live it all the time?" was asked.

I grinned broadly. "Of course not. I'm human just like everyone else here. I find myself out with friends and we go out for dinner and I overeat. And you know, it's ok. I get up the next morning and get right back on that horse. I don't beat myself up over cheese fries the night before, I look forward to a good day of managing my health. And that's an important thing. With any diet, with any program, give yourself a break. Take a day for you. One day a week or one meal a week, just eat whatever you want and don't look back. If you want the Chinese buffet that day, do it. If you want a huge Reuben, have it. Who wants to go through life day after day denying yourself some of the good things in life which aren't necessarily all that good for you? If I tell you here and now that you can't ever have chocolate again, what's going to happen? That's right, in about three hours, all you'll be able to think about is chocolate and how much you love it and you'll never be able to have it again. You'll find chocolate is the sole focus of your life before the end of the day and you'll put down a large Hershey bar before bed. That's just how we are, how we're wired as humans. So, don't deny yourself food you like, just go easy on everything and pay attention to what you eat.

Is that advice doctor approved? Nutritionist approved? Certified Diabetes Educator approved? Absolutely.

Here, again, the advice is to be sensible. Sure, I have pizza now and then, just not a entire large meat lover's with extra cheese. I may still order the large, but I've come to love Mediterranean and veggie pizzas and I try to eat two or three slices instead of killing it off in one sitting. In my desk drawer at work, I keep small, individually wrapped chocolate blocks and I eat one whenever I want. Instead of taking it down in two bites, I take little mouse nibbles off it and let the chocolate melt on my tongue. That way I get ten or twelve minutes of chocolate pleasure instead of ninety seconds. Stop and enjoy the experience, prolong it, live in the moment. No, I don't live it every single minute of the day, but living the plan eighty or ninety percent of the time is eighty or ninety percent more than I used to.

Live your life, but love you in the process."

Chapter 24

October 2006

I went with friends one Saturday morning in the crisp mountain air to Bass Lake in Blowing Rock, North Carolina. There was still mist hanging in low spots on the Blue Ridge Parkway. My friends wanted to walk around the lake then walk up to the manor house up on the hill, tour it, and look back down into the valley below. I decided to walk the mountain trail.

We parked and got out and went through the wood gate lined entrance. My friends started walking around Bass Lake, but I peeled off to the right and started jogging down the mountain trail in a zipped up garnet fleece jacket. I jogged for a couple of hundred yards downhill until the gravel roadbed turned up and right into a steep incline. I dropped to a walk and continued around the road that wound around the mountain. When the road flattened out a bit, I jogged, then dropped back into a walk when the incline grew too steep. As I warmed up, I had to unzip my fleece jacket. I passed riders on horseback coming back down the mountain and joggers passed me as I continued up the road. I found a good walking pace and maintained it.

The leaves were just into turning their colors for the fall with the peak of brilliance coming in a few weeks. I was never one to care about leaf colors, but the canopy of trees covered and insulated the trail and I could reach out and touch the branches as I made my way. The trees insulated the trail from the outside world, both light and sound. The road was darker than the outside world from the trees crowding in and noise was isolated to the crunching of my running shoes on dirt and gravel and my breathing. I was alone in the woods on a mountain road walking and jogging to the top.

After half an hour, the road began to open up into a larger area with a barn and wagons. I passed tourists sitting on wooden benches as I rounded a corner to see down into the valley. I had made it to the top of the mountain and could see the huge, white manor house and the lake below. I stopped and surveyed all that was laid out before me in the lush valley surrounded by miles of green forest. The view was amazing and I stood there for a few minutes just taking in the panorama of color and beauty there on the mountaintop. Then I pulled off my fleece jacket, tied the arms around my waist, and started jogging down the trail.

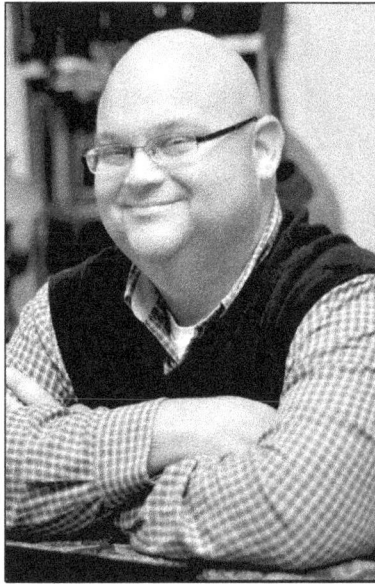

Carl Eugene Moore, MBA, MFA

…holds an MBA in Accounting & Finance, an MBA in Health Care Management, an MFA in Creative Writing, and is currently doing his doctoral work in Health Administration with a focus on Health Informatics and Health Care Quality. He has poetry, fiction, nonfiction, and photography published and is currently the nonfiction editor for a literary magazine and a feature editor for an academic journal. He teaches graduate and undergraduate courses in Health and Medical Informatics and English.

carlmoore@yahoo.com | www.carlmoore.org

passingthroughbook.wordpress.com